**Green Body
Green Birth**

# Green Body
# Green Birth

A Revolutionary Guide for
Preconception, Pregnancy, and Birth

Mary Oscategui

The information contained herein reflects only the opinion of Mary Oscategui. In no way is it to be considered medical or product advice. Specific medical advice should be obtained from a licensed health care practitioner. Consult with your doctor before you begin any fitness, exercise, nutrition, diet, weight loss, heart attack or stroke risk reduction program or other change in lifestyle. This information is in no way meant to treat, cure or prevent any disease or illness from happening.

Mary Oscategui, has provided this book and the information on it for consumer education purposes only. Therefore, you should consult with your personal physician or other health-care professional if you have any healthcare related questions or before embarking on a new diet or fitness program. If a medical problem appears or persists, do not disregard or delay seeking medical advice from your personal physician or other qualified healthcare provider based on something you read in the book. Accordingly, Mary Oscategui, expressly disclaims any liability, loss, damage, or injury caused by information contained in this book.

Mention of specific companies, organizations, or authorities in this book does not imply endorsement by the author or publisher, nor does mention of specific companies, organizations, or authorities imply their endorsement of this book, its author, or the publisher.

Internet addresses were accurate at the time this book went to press.

Library of Congress Cataloging-in-Publication has been applied for.

Copyright © 2012, Mary Oscategui

All rights reserved. No part of this book may be reproduced, stored, or transmitted by any means—whether auditory, graphic, mechanical, or electronic—without written permission of both publisher and author, except in the case of brief excerpts used in critical articles and reviews. Unauthorized reproduction of any part of this work is illegal and is punishable by law.

ISBN 978-0-615-55112-8

*For Bella Luna & Taj Orion Sky*

# Acknowledgments

A deep heartfelt gratitude to all my past, current, and future teachers and for the following people and organizations who have deeply influenced my life:

My mom, my dad, my beautiful moon: Bella Luna, my soon to be born son: Taj Orion Sky, my children's father, my sister, my brother, my midwives: Mary Jackson and Diane Holzer, my birth doulas: Cheryl Clearwater and Samantha Stormer, Ray Castellino, Troy Casey, Paul Chek, Ken Cook, Michael Green, Alexandra Zissu, Molly Arthur, Emily Schaffer, Shea Anne, Eckhart Tolle, Wayne Dyer, Don Miguel Ruiz, Lao Tzu, Joseph Campbell, Dr Bruce Lipton, Dr Candice Pert, Dr Daniel Amen, Penney Pierce, Krishnamurti, EWG, Center for Environmental Health, Healthy Child Healthy World, Center for Children's Health & the Environment, Council on Environmental Health, Institute for Children's Environmental Health, WHO Children's Environmental Health, Agency for Toxic Substances & Disease Registry, The Natural Child Project, Every Mother Counts, Coalition for Improving Maternity Services, Children's Health Environmental Coalition, Green Child Magazine, Kiwi Magazine, International Maternity Institute and, IMI Greenproofers and Greenbirth Educators.

# Contents

| | |
|---|---|
| Introduction | xiii |
| Green What Does It Mean? | 1 |
| The Discovery | 7 |
| Toxins | 11 |
| Green Body Green Birth 4 R's | 19 |
| We Are One: Parts of a Whole System | 27 |
| Preconception | 59 |
| Pregnancy | 75 |
| Birth & Postpartum | 87 |
| Conclusion | 103 |
| Green Body Green Birth Spotlight: Troy Casey | 107 |
| The Story of EcoBirth | 115 |
| Resources | 155 |

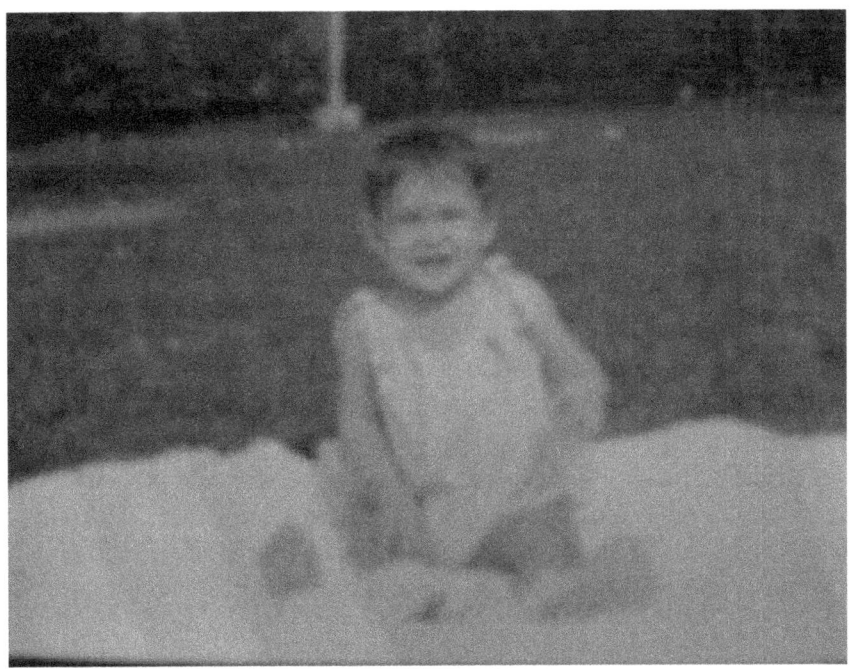

# Introduction

As I began my journey, what started out to be a standard book about greenproofing, blossomed into something much deeper. In the world of maternity and green, it seems that pretty much every day a new article or headline crosses the screen or cover of the newspaper which gives rise to various fears surrounding pregnancy, the environment, and our health. In watching this in myself and my clients, I felt an urgency to empower us all to regain a sense of peace through a more balanced perspective on our body and the environment. I also felt a strong need to address the specific pressures and fears that arise as one enters the green movement.

As a mother, I feel an infinite responsibility to myself and the world that I will leave behind to my children and the generations to come. While writing this book, I felt the greatest gift I could offer in service to expecting families, couples trying to conceive, and new parents, was to provide a balanced perspective with healthy, practical oriented solutions through an understanding of the seamless connection between our bodies, minds, and the environment.

Such understanding may provide you a tremendous potential opening, which can awaken within you a freedom that can deeply change your life, your relationship to the world, and your children. May this book be an inspiration and a guide toward that intention.

About the book:

Being that there are so many amazing green books already out there covering the world of toxic chemicals, environments, products and green lifestyle options around us, I felt compelled to offer a different perspective on green, drawing our attention inward specifically focusing on greening our body's environment. I write this book as a woman, an expecting mom, mother, and friend. Although I have a wealth of education, experience, and credentials behind me, I am not a scientist or doctor. My intention is not to preach to you or try to convince you to follow what I have discovered works for me, or back up every point with a scientific document. My intention is to share my deepest heartfelt passion for what has spoken through me and my most important discoveries. I encourage all my readers to do their own research, experiment, question everything, and find out what works best for them.

A bit about myself:

The world first welcomed me in the Big Apple. I grew up in a one bedroom apartment in a family of five in Astoria, Queens New York. Both my parents were immigrants who worked very hard to live the American dream. My mother sacrificed everything she could to provide me with the best education available and my father always reminded me to dig deeper in order learn the facts from all sides. I attended Catholic school during the week and Sunday school on church days. I remained in Catholic School until college. My mother was a born again Evangelical Christian and my father was a Unitarian. My father and I had many deep conversations about a variety of religions and he had a fairly inclusive perspective of spirituality. I am so grateful to both of them as this variety of diverse perspectives and belief systems has kept my mind open to all and it is through the vehicle of education and the exposure to these diverse perspectives that has turned out to be my life's calling and passion.

My not-so-green history:

I was born naturally but in a hospital setting, given every vaccine available and recommended for children at the time, and administered every antibiotic when sick. Unknowingly, my mom also used the most toxic household cleaners available on the market when cleaning our home. She also collected a ton of fragrances via perfumes on her dresser drawer. Although we ate mostly non-processed foods, our food was not organic. On the other hand, you could not find any junk food lying around our house unless it was one of our birthdays once a year. My father enjoyed growing alfalfa sprouts in our kitchen cupboards and made us fresh, carrot, celery, and apple juice just about every morning. In my late teens I was led to an educational path of health, fitness, and nutrition which greatly impacted my life's calling and awakening. I feel very blessed with my life's path.

Today:

When looking back at my life, I know that both my parents did the best they could and with what they knew. I consider it a tremendous blessing that after all the pleasures and pains I experienced so far throughout my lifetime, I stand here before you today empowered with a joy for life and living and at peace knowing every moment is a gift. I am extremely thankful for every struggle, challenge, and roadblock that has come my way as they all have been the most significant blessings and opportunities in my life. I am also appreciative for the opportunity to experience birth in its most natural form. 18 hours of labor at home without drugs and a 9lb baby girl taught me a lot about the strength, intelligence, and the capacity my body has to push through challenges, physical and otherwise.

As strange as it may sound, I am also very grateful to have experienced all the stresses, anxieties, and fears surrounding a single mother's responsibility to raise a daughter while trying to maintain the "I can do it all" mantra that has been so looked up to in our society. Now being pregnant with my second child and running a maternity institution, I have learned how easy it can be to feel overwhelmed, fearful, and anxious with all the conflicting information, possible dangers lurking below the surface, and all the judgments swirling around the choices a woman makes for her pregnancy and her birth. All of this has just empowered me all the more.

I dedicate this book to all those who have a deep interest in establishing a healthy and balanced perspective of their body and of the world. I also dedicated this book to all the pre-conceiving parents, expecting parents, new parents, babies, children, teenagers, maternity professionals, eco-consultants, and those in the green movement at large who are truly seeking to leave behind a better world for all beings.

## *[Green]: What does it mean?*

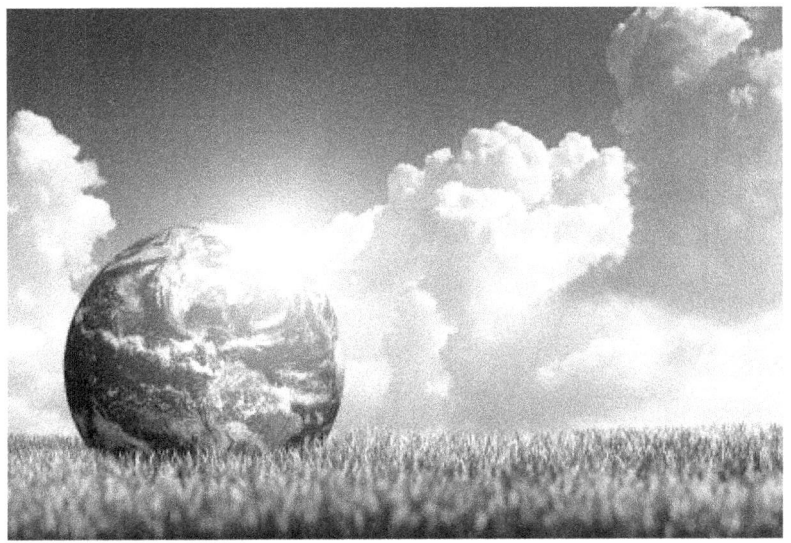

Whenever I am talking with a friend, colleague, working with a new client, or teaching new students I like to explore the word "green" and ask what it means to them. I have found that this is such a relevant component and starting point before initiating any kind of steps toward a green lifestyle.

Green can mean different things to different people and sometimes perceptions can lead to assumptions that can easily hinder us from inviting the opportunity to contribute to the sustainability of our lives, humanity, all of life and our earth.

How most people define what green means to them really depends on how they have first been exposed to the concept in the media and their community. This initially happens through articles, advertisements, campaigns, commercials, petitions, and so on.

## For some Green can mean:

- An environmental movement
- Conservation
- Consuming less
- Sustainability
- Clean energy, food, air, and water
- Environmentally-friendly
- Saving the environment
- Reduce, reuse, recycle, restore
- Reducing our impact on the planet
- Simple living
- Prevention of toxic exposures
- Tree hugger
- Expensive

**Additional words and symbols that have also been associated with the word "Green":**
- Fertility
- Nature
- Healing

- Greenhouse
- Well-Being Balance
- 4$^{th}$ Chakra: Heart Chakra
- Envy/Jealousy
- Growth
- Calming
- Refreshing
- Money/Wealth

**For the purposes of this book, the term green will be used to understand and connect with the environment of your body in the forms of:**

- Health
- Safety
- Nourishment
- Balance
- Sustainability of Life
- Consuming Less
- Fertility
- Pregnancy
- Birth
- Renewal
- Healing
- Reducing, Reusing, Recycling, Restoring

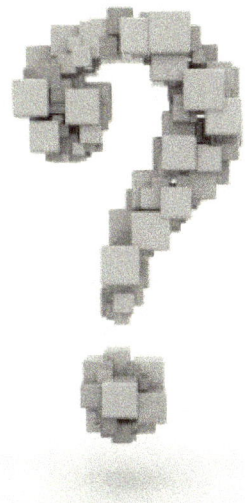

Whether you are just starting on a green journey or consider yourself a green veteran, the following questions can be wonderful ways to affirm and connect with what green means for you. These questions may also help strengthen your drive and commitment towards developing a green lifestyle. Experiment and reflect with your own questions as well so that you can more clearly understand your motives for going green and/or maintaining a green lifestyle.

- What does going green mean to you? You may be familiar what it means for others and our society, but what does it mean specifically for you?
- Use your notepad or journal to write the words or things come to mind when you think of the term green.
- Is going green important to you? Why?
- Does green living inspire you? How?
- Does green living challenge you? How so?
- Do you feel empowered by living a green lifestyle? If so, in what ways?
- Why do you think some people are turned off by the green movement?
- Is there anything that turns you off about the green movement? [Describe]

# *The Discovery*

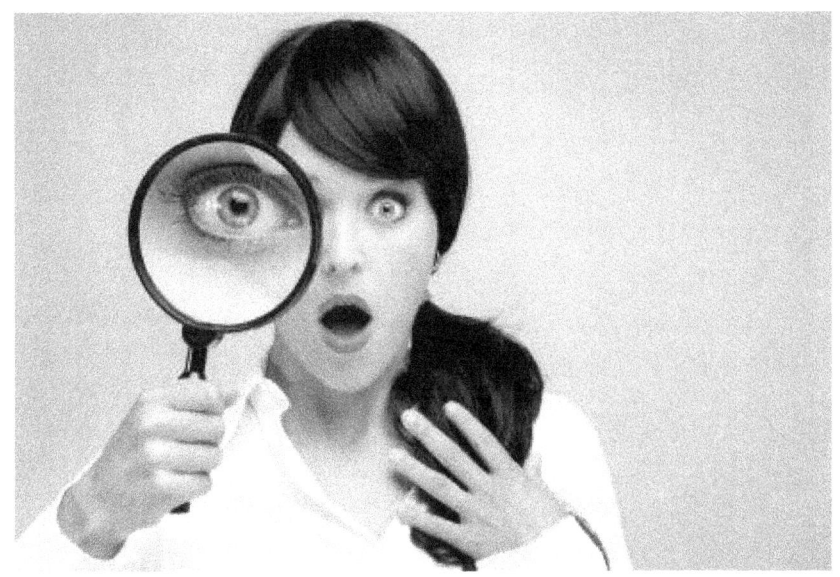

When starting on green journey and understanding what green means specifically to you, there comes what is called The Discovery Stage. This is the stage where one becomes excited about the discovery of new information, but this is also the state when fear, anger or frustration arises, and sometimes one feels a loss of power or control. These disturbing emotions usually arise when discovering that one has been misled, misinformed, or discovering that you have fallen for propaganda of some sort. This is also known as "Greenwashing", a marketing tactic of misleading consumers about a product or service's environmental friendliness.

A 2010 study by TerraChoice, an independent testing and certification organization revealed out of 5,296 products only 265 were really as green as they claimed. 95% of "green" products are being greenwashed.

Going through this stage of discovery may be particularly challenging for just about anyone but in particular it can be difficult for a woman who is pregnant or recently became a mother. Her body and mind have already undergone many physical and emotional changes, and now she has to deal with handling all this new information regarding the various dangers lurking in her cupboards, her air, her breast milk, her food, her furnishings, her car, her supermarket, and her baby's world and add to that the great possibility of being misled.

I have worked with so many pregnant women and mothers who are excited about beginning their green journey only to become quickly disenchanted with feelings of disappointment, guilt, fear, and even anger.

How can we best deal with these feelings? Are they valid? The first step is to acknowledge them as normal and healthy. When discovering such information, it is perfectly natural to have some kind of emotional reaction. During this discovery phase, rather than moving forward and understanding the opportunity that lies in front of us, many of us get stuck in our feelings and sense of helplessness.

Where to Begin?
- Acknowledge your feelings
- In every challenge, lies an opportunity. Find your opportunity.

- Focus on a practical plan of action keeping in mind that trying to achieve perfection is not realistic or practical.
- Start with simple baby steps
- Know your sources and resources. There are many great tools and resources available. For example: Good Guide (goodguide.com), The Safe Cosmetics Database (safecosmetics.org), Healthy Child Healthy World (healthychild.org), and The Environmental Working Group (ewg.org)
- Get into the habit of asking questions about everything you are putting into your body, on your body, and what is surrounding you.
- Vote with Your Dollars
- Ask for Support
- Surround yourself with people, places, and things that inspire you and give you hope.
- Get active and involved with your community.
- Collaborate with others who share your concerns, passion, and goals.
- Invite space and reflection

## *TOXINS*

## Toxic Free

Most of us who pursue a green lifestyle, strive to be toxic-free, but is striving to be toxic-free, a realistic goal? It's a question I continue to ask myself and challenge you to as well; as I find that the world of toxins is not so black and white. Perhaps it's not so much about striving to be toxic-free as it is about understanding how toxins work, managing them, reducing them to a minimum, and ending our support and contribution to their spread in our environment.

What is a toxin?

A toxin can be a chemical which occurs naturally or synthetically. Toxins can come from a biological origin, also known as Biotoxins, or toxins can come from an environmental origin, known as Environmental toxins. Environmental toxins can sometimes explicitly include contaminants that are man-made.

According to Wikipedia:

*When used non-technically, the term "toxin" is often applied to any toxic substance. Toxic substances not directly of biological origin are also termed poisons.*

*In the context of alternative medicine the term is often used to refer to any substance claimed to cause ill health, ranging anywhere from trace amounts of pesticides to common food items like refined sugar or additives such as monosodium glutamate (MSG).*

Pamela Duff RN, CNSC, author of *Nature's Pharmacy* explains the basics of toxins,

> **A toxin** *is simply a poison that can affect the body by internal or external means. A toxin can be a chemical which occurs naturally or in synthetic form. More than 120,000 human-made chemicals have been introduced into the environment, in one form or another and this number continues to grow each year at a phenomenal rate. At the same time, microbial toxins, being influenced by the vast numbers of chemicals, are mutating beyond belief. Each category of microbes produces species that generates*

*toxins in host cells. Evidence is proving a definitive link between the accumulation of toxins in body tissues and the development of chronic diseases. External toxins, either chemical or microbial, enter the body through food, water, air, or physical contact with the skin or mucous membranes. Internal toxins, as the free radicals, are produced inside the body through normal metabolic processes or through the decomposition of foods in the small and large intestines. Bacterial toxins and yeast overgrowth can also form in cases of chronic constipation.*

*Under normal circumstances, the body is able to eliminate toxins from the body via urine, feces, exhalation, and perspiration. Thus, the major organs involved in elimination are the kidneys, liver, colon, lungs, and skin. In addition, WBCs (white blood cells) of the immune system are designed to neutralize microbial toxins. The liver is the organ primarily responsible for breaking toxins into harmless byproducts, which are eliminated into the stool or through the kidneys into the urine.*

*The process of elimination can be hampered for one reason or another. When a particular toxin overwhelms the normal excretion mechanisms, the body produces inflammation in the area of the toxin trying to rid itself of the problem. These inflammatory areas signal the start of a disease. They are actually signals the body is sending, stating that it cannot rid itself of accumulating toxins. If the toxins remain, the body then moves into the next stage, where they are deposited in areas where they will do the least harm. These areas are usually fat cells, cysts, polyps or tumors. After years of storage, the toxins move into body cells and tissues. They ultimately produce such degenerative diseases as cancer, diabetes, arthritis, and heart disease."*

When most of us think of toxins (poisons), our immediate reaction is to fear or avoid them. This is an initial healthy response as we have an innate protective mechanism for the purpose of our survival.

Nature also strives to survive and as a result has developed its own protective mechanisms via toxins. For example:

- Many plants are highly poisonous when ingested and even simply touching certain plant species can also be a serious health hazard. Plants contain a host of toxins to

- protect themselves from predators, including some of the plants that have become staples in modern civilization.
- Molds themselves produce some of the most potent toxins known to man. Thousands of people each year have their health greatly affected by mold infestations in their homes. In times past viruses were blamed for many health problems that molds are now being blamed for. A recent study in the Lancet suggested that perhaps 90% of sinus infections are fungal related.
- The largest polluter in America is not a factory or a corporation, but is in fact a volcano. Kilauea on the Big Island of Hawaii produces as much smog as the twelve largest factories in America combined. The volcanic smog known as "vog" has disrupted the lives and caused severe health problems for many thousands of people living on the Big Island and nearby islands. The number one air polluter in the state of Washington over the last decade was a volcano as well—Mt St Helens. In 2004, and 2005 Mt St Helens was producing around 50-250 tons of sulfur dioxide per day. All of the state's industries combined produced about 120 tons a day.

## Man Made Toxins

Humans also produce many toxins not only within themselves, but also in our environment which has contributed to the pollution and extinction of certain species. For example:

- For our survival: some of us may resort to the use of pesticides, exterminators, or exterminating products to get rid of rodents, insects, pests, etc…
- For our pleasure or convenience: We over consume, we toss our waste away into the ocean and landfills and streams, we smoke cigarettes and expose others through second hand smoke, we burn our garbage and industrial waste and pollute the air with toxic substances, we put toxic fragrances on our body and force others to breathe it, we drink alcohol to intoxicate ourselves, etc.

- For profit: Certain companies have made it a common practice to profit from the production and manufacturing of products, pesticides, and a variety of chemicals that are known to be toxic.

According to the 2010 annual national analysis of the Toxics Release Inventory (TRI) via The U.S. Environmental Protection Agency (EPA), 3.93 billion pounds of toxic chemicals were released into the environment nationwide, a 16 percent increase from 2009, however a decrease from the 6.16 billion pounds of toxic chemicals released on- and off-site in 2001.

This data does not include toxic emissions from cars, trucks, sources of pesticides, volatile organic compounds, or other non-industrial sources.

## Greenwashing

As introduced in the previous chapter, *The Discovery*, the practice known as "Greenwashing" is becoming more and more common as most companies are jumping on the bandwagon to appear earth conscious and 'green'. The term 'sustainability' has also become watered down and you will find all sorts of companies using the term when most of these companies have virtually nothing to do with biological sustainability whatsoever. Only a very small fraction of companies have actually taken real steps toward true sustainability. If a business is not moving toward actual sustainability, one has to question whether it can really be considered green.

As a result of these blurry lines, we are now starting to see certifying bodies become more common place to provide regulations and standards. Greenguard, USDA Organic, Energy Star, Fair Trade Certified, Green Seal Certified, Rainforest Alliance, and the BPI Compostable are a few of many that are leading the way forward.

## Fear and Anger

Fear is the most common tactic that has been used in our society both intentionally and unintentionally as a means to instantly persuade oneself or another to change their behavior by joining a movement, opposing a movement, buying a product, avoiding a product, joining a religion, opposing a religion, accepting a theory, rejecting a theory, supporting a political party, opposing a political party, and so on. As a result fear tactics are commonly used in marketing and can lead some to feelings of anger.

According to Dictionary.com:
*Fear is a distressing emotion aroused by impending danger, evil, pain, etc., whether the threat is real or imagined; also, the feeling or condition of being afraid.*

*Anger is a strong feeling of displeasure and belligerence aroused by a wrong; wrath; etc.*

Perhaps we could consider fear and anger as psychological toxins since they can have many physical and mental consequences. As a result, I question whether fear or anger, being toxins themselves, are the best solutions to perceive or deal with the influx of toxic substances overwhelmingly entering our lives and environment. I encourage you to examine whether fear or anger, beyond the initial instinctual reaction, is really beneficial to deal with our physical and environmental problems.

As human beings we have been faced with challenges of all kinds for many millions of years and yet humans have always found a way to distinguish between a poisonous berry and a non-poisonous berry; the only difference today being that we have a lot more "berries" to distinguish.

Perspective is everything and I believe when dealing with toxins of any kind, it is a matter of remaining aware, staying educated, adapting to changes in our environment, and getting involved and active with ourselves and within our community. Only once we understand the bigger picture can we take the appropriate action and be responsible.

What can you do when a fear or anger about toxins sets in?
- Empower yourself with an attitude toward education and solutions.
- Question everything. Investigate. Don't just take someone's word for it, especially if they are selling something.

- Know your sources and resources.
- Take responsibility for your choices and actions.
- Never underestimate the power of voting with your dollar. Every dollar you spend creates a supply/demand ripple that can easily be measured and felt. We can't expect that non-green companies will begin to care for the environment when we are still purchasing their products. In fact every time you purchase their product you are literally saying "don't change; I want this just as it is".
- Buy organic. Buy local. Buy sustainable.
- Simply your life and eliminate those things (big and small) that aren't truly needed for your health and well-being.
- Get active with your local community.
- Share ideas and work together with one another to come up with solutions and advocate for change.

Understanding our toxins: internally, externally, biologically and environmentally are essential. It is up to us to stop contributing and supporting our own and others' man-made toxins. These changes are very powerful and will not only contribute to the sustainability of ourselves and our planet, but they also mean thousands of extra dollars in the hands of those who are investing in the sustainable and green movements.

# The 4 R's of Green Body Green Birth

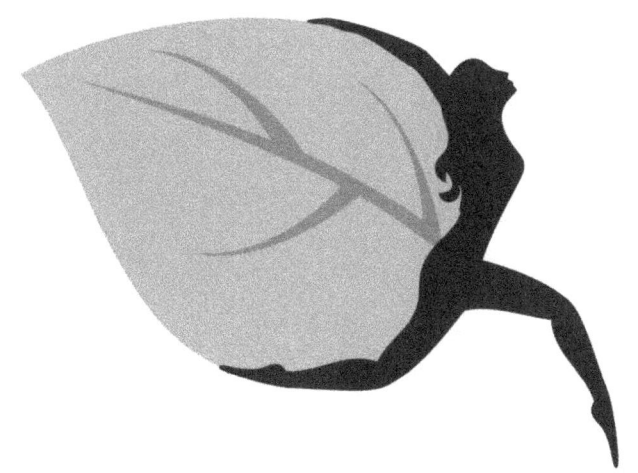

Just as you'll find the 4 R's of waste management in our outer environment, Green Body Green Birth has come up with 4 R's for our body's environment.

By supporting and encouraging the healthy sustainability of our own human body, we have a much greater opportunity to thrive and contribute to the health and sustainability of our earth.

In the same way, this kind of symbiotic relationship happens between a mom and her baby. When mom supports and encourages the health and sustainability of her body, she supports and encourages the health and sustainability of her baby. The two are one entity. This is obvious to all when the baby is in the womb, but it becomes less obvious to some as the child grows, yet the two always remain one. The mother not only imparts her genes to the child, but her nutrients, her bacteria, her consciousness: her movements, her habits and everything else.

## The 4R's of Green Body Green Birth:

### 1. Reduce.

Just as we commit ourselves to reducing the amount of waste we produce in our outer environment, we can take charge and do the same for our minds and bodies.

The majority of adults and children in our mainstream society are not just suffering from physical obesity but mental obesity as well. According to the World Health Organization, obesity has reached epidemic proportions globally, with at least 2.8 million people dying each year as a result of being overweight or obese and childhood obesity is one of the most serious public health challenges of the 21st century.

In addition, I believe we are also experiencing a mental obesity, where our minds have become overweight and dependent on constant stimulus 24/7, from working, television, ipads, smartphones, computers, movies, radio, video games, magazines, twitter, facebook, iphone apps, and much more. It seems like everything is speeding up. The space between thoughts and images and between ads we see have grown smaller.

Like obesity of the body, obesity of the mind can pose many health issues from depression to ADHD to sleep disorders.

According to Roots of Action, in 1970, the average age at which children watched television was four years old. Today, the average age is four months. The typical child before the age of five is watching 4 ½ hours of television per day, 40% of their waking hours!

We can reduce mental noise, stress, waste, and information overload by inviting space. This can be done by spending less time accumulating more information and more time in meditation, yoga, hiking, nature, or just by simply resting.

On a physical level, we can commit to only consuming that which is needed for our body. Excess food consumption leads to excess waste in the body, and it leads to an inefficient human machine. A weak body necessitates an entire system and economy to care for it.

## 2. Reuse what is sustainable and nourishing for the mind, body, and soul.

How often do we catch ourselves reusing or repeating negative thoughts, negative physical habits or perhaps re-entering into unhealthy relationships?

A powerful way to transform our lives is by reusing what is nourishing our bodies, minds, and souls. Set aside a small time each day to remind yourself of what nourishes you, what it is that you enjoy, what feels good to you and who feels good to you.

Just as we can easily create bad habits, we can also reshape them into good ones that we can continue to reuse. Reusing what internally sustains us prevents accumulation of waste within us setting us on a path of sustainable relationships and a sustainable life.

Below are a few simple ways and examples to reuse what sustains and nourishes you. Experiment or try what works best for you:

- Spend more time with the people in your life that inspire you or feel good to be around.
- Reuse your own nourishing thoughts and of those who are living the lifestyle you truly aspire to.
- Take reflective walks a few minutes each day
- Dance
- Sing

- Play
- Relax
- Listen to your favorite motivational speaker
- Meditate or participate in restorative yoga

**3. Recycle or transmute your body and/or your story.**

*Your Body:*

The body is a recycling machine. It is constantly recycling proteins, hormones, nutrients, waste, and transmuting excess consumption into storage. It's time to transmute all that extra storage and waste into energy in order to create a new body, and new shape, and a new life. All the junk food or excess carbs that are now hanging on your body, weighing you down, can literally become the fuel to propel you into a new life.

By nourishing your body with locally grown organic non-processed foods, engaging in a daily form of balanced exercise, getting more sunshine, getting more deep sleep, reducing your stress, and hydrating with clean natural water and fresh fruit juices, you will help your body to remove toxins, clean the pipes, and burn up all that accumulated fuel hanging around you like dead weight.

*Your Story:*

We each have a story about the world and about ourselves that affects our actions, choices, decisions, personalities, and so on. Stories can be limiting. For some of us, our story can hold us back from thriving or achieving our greatest human potential. Most of these stories don't serve or sustain us, nor do they give us an opportunity to invite our highest self or our deepest impulses and deepest heart longings.

These stories get recycled over and over. It's time to stop recycling these limiting concepts of who we are. Let go of them completely and only recycle the most unlimited thoughts we can think, feel, and imagine. Only your highest and most nurturing thoughts should be recycled.

An example of how to do this is to evaluate and assess your current story followed by inviting your dream story or your vision. You may start by asking yourself the following questions:

How do you currently feel about yourself? How would you describe yourself? How would others describe you? What do you like about yourself? What don't you like about yourself? What are your strengths? What do you have to offer the world? If you had the ability to accomplish anything, what would it be? What is your dream story or vision? What would your dream story look and feel like? Who would be in it?

The next step would be to make it happen! Plan, prepare, and take action. Invite practical and realistic ways to make your dream story or vision happen. Take baby steps. It does not need to happen overnight. Every small step you take paves the way, guides you into a new direction, and invites your dream or vision to become a reality.

### 4. Recover/Restore what has been broken inside of you

*A Time to Heal, Restore, and Renew:*

This is my personal favorite of the 4R's and I feel a largely overlooked or avoided component.

Many of us of are lucky if we have anytime in our today for just the tiniest bit of space. Some of our lives may reflect the following:

Wake up at 6:30am, dress and feed and our children, dress and feed ourselves, rush to work, work until 5pm, come home and feed and care for our children, return some phone calls, catch up with our friends, check emails, check the latest news stories on the web, check Facebook posts, check Twitter…..all this in addition to the periodic doctors appointments, dentist appointments, mechanic appointments, calling the plumber, walks with the dog, grocery shopping, eating meals, going to the bathroom, brushing teeth, doing make up, paying bills, paying taxes, planning birthday parties, going to birthday parties, going to school events, cleaning the house, cleaning the car, doing laundry, and much more.

As I shared with Green Body Green Birth's $1^{st}$ R: Reduce, space opens up when we minimize the amount of noise, stress, information, and activity going in and around us.

When space opens up, a new world unfolds. Stored up emotions, traumas, unnoticed observations, creativity, intuition, and clarity, all rise to the surface.

Quite often in our society we are taught to suppress our emotions and to avoid them if we can. In addition, when we are too busy to deal with our emotions and frustrations, or suppress them, they may show up later as a physical ailment in our body. Suppressed emotions may take form in the shape of depression, arthritis, cancer, and sometimes even death. Many scientists, doctors, and researchers have dedicated their lives to understanding the connection between our emotions, thoughts, beliefs and their impact on our physical body. Dr Bruce Lipton, Dr Candace Pert, and Dr Daniel Amen are just a few of many who have contributed greatly to this understanding. There is also a field in medicine known as Psychosomatic Medicine.

Wikipedia defines psychosomatic medicine as:
- An interdisciplinary medical field studying the relationships of social, psychological, and behavioral factors on bodily processes and quality of life in humans and animals.
- The influence that the mind has over physical processes — including the manifestations of disabilities that are based on intellectual infirmities, rather than actual injuries or physical limitations — is manifested in treatment by phrases such as the **power of suggestion**, the use of "positive thinking" and concepts like "mind over matter".

As mentioned earlier in the book, many who begin their journey toward sustainability and health may be met with feelings of anger, guilt, fear, anxiety or depression. Our first instinct may be to push away these feelings, ignore, them, or fall deeper into them. I believe it is vital to take such an opportunity to welcome these feelings, discover their roots, and allow them to move through us and out of us so we may heal, restore, and renew ourselves. This is a key step towards well-being. I also believe it is important to allow time to heal and as we go through the healing process, surrounding ourselves with supportive environments and people. There are also many great retreats all over the country (and the world) where space and healing is given priority. Retreats can be profound and can be that catalyst that forever breaks your old patterns.

# *We Are One:*
# *Parts of a Whole System*

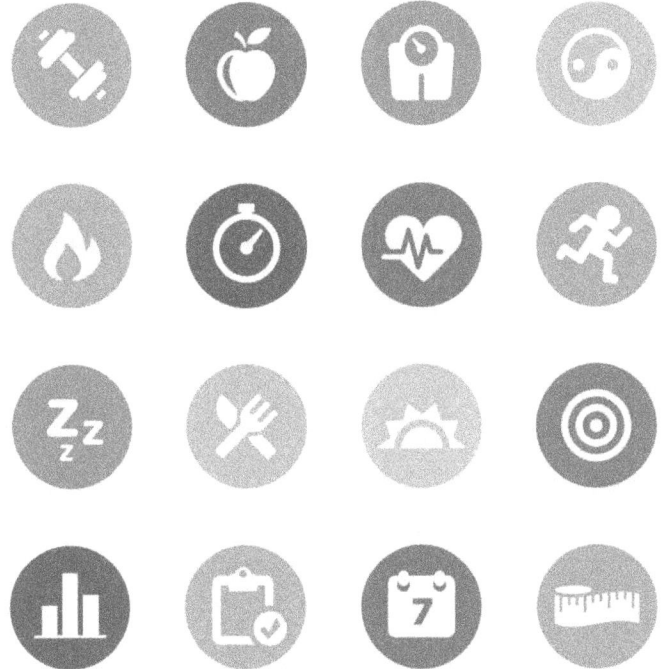

*"Healthy Me = a Healthy Planet"*
*~ Certified Health Nut, Troy Casey*

***Green Body Green Birth's #1 Protective Device* from toxins and disease is a healthy body.** Although we can all do our best to prepare and prevent toxic exposure outside of us, the best prevention begins inside, with our health. By caring for our body and strengthening the immune system, our body can be better equipped to handle the toxins around us. If our body is overburdened with toxins from within, it can't sufficiently handle the toxins without. In addition, when we feel lethargic, weak, or are too busy trying to deal with our own health problems, how can we be prepared to give, get active, and work together with one another as a society to initiate change?

In this chapter, we are going to take a look at what keeps us and our earth thriving.

Most often we attribute the cause of disease, and the cure to disease to one major factor depending on the latest information that has entered our brains. We have developed an A to Z mentality. The cure for A is such and such. The cure for B is such and such. However the more we understand how intricately related all diseases and cures are, the more it becomes evident that it is not just one thing causing imbalance— it is a bit of everything.

How many times have you read a book or article about toxins in the environment, or one about candida, or mercury, or exercise, or diet, or stress, or sleep, or nutrition, or parasites, and immediately become convinced that this one factor is the cause of ALL disease and ALL your aches and pains? Of course what usually happens is that a couple months later you read another book or article and become convinced that some other factor is the 'big one', and is 'definitely' the missing link and the cure for everything. It's amazing how many missing links there are—an infinite number it seems!

In order for us to function our best and contribute our best to the world around us, the following spectrum of components are necessary to support optimal functioning and sustainability of our body and our environment:

- Air
- Water
- Food
- Sunshine
- Exercise/Movement

- Emotions/Thoughts
- Sleep/Restoration
- Stress Management
- Energy
- Environment
- Intuition
- Balance

## Air

The air we breathe and how we breathe are both very important. In Chinese Medicine, breathe or prana is also linked our life force. There is no question that we should pay attention and stand up for clean air in our environment, however, our bodies would benefit tremendously with the same kind of awareness and attention to how we breathe. After all, breathe is the one essential component of living that we can live the least amount of time without.

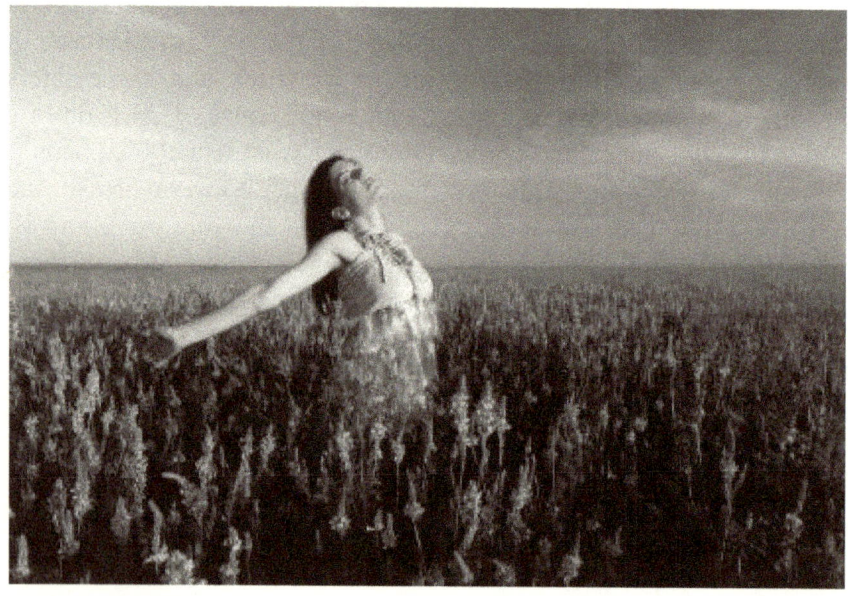

According to dancer and teacher Michelle Ava "Proper breathing has profound effects on our health. Over 70 percent of waste by-products are eliminated through our breathing and our skin.

When our blood is heavily oxygenated it becomes very difficult for virus and bacteria to grow."

Let's look at some of the common ways people breathe and their effects.
- Shallow Breathing (Chest) vs. Diaphragmatic Breathing (Belly)
- Reverse Breathing

### Shallow Breathing

Shallow Breathe, also known as chest breathing, limits our breathing capacity to the lungs and upper thoracic area whereas diaphragmatic breathe, considered the healthiest way to breathe, allows oxygen to travel deeply into the lungs and abdomen. We are all born diaphragmatically breathing, but overtime, due to a variety of reasons like stress, poor posture, poor habits, fast-paced lifestyle, etc...., we become conditioned to a more shallow breathe.

Shallow breathing is actually more common that you might think. Often times this shows up as mouth breathing.

According to the researchers at normalbreathing.com,

"Over 90% of modern people suffer from **breathing problems**. The common problems include chest breathing, mouth breathing, and hyperventilation (increased minute ventilation). All these abnormalities reduce **oxygen levels** in body cells and promote chronic diseases. We can find solid medical evidence testifying that sick people have too heavy automatic breathing (hyperventilation) at rest."

The researchers go onto say, "When seeing modern people on Western streets and in public places, one may easily notice that up to 30-40% of them can breathe through their mouths when walking or even while standing or sitting. Most people these days are mouth breathers. The same can be easily observed during night sleep. Some decades ago mouth breathing was socially abnormal and unacceptable. However, it is very common these days. In adults, mouth breathing causes advance of many chronic diseases, including sleep apnea, snoring at night, morning fatigue, dry mouth syndrome, headache, morning fatigue (or morning headache fatigue) and other symptoms. Children mouth breathing (especially during sleep), as well as in infants, toddlers and older children, are new health problems that promote chronic diseases, including frequent infections, asthma, rashes, diathesis, bed wetting, etc. However, for a healthy person, nose breathing should be the norm 24-7."

## Reverse Breathing

There is also what is referred to reverse breathing. Reverse breathing happens when during inhalation instead of your chest and abdomen expanding outward, your chest and abdomen draw inward. When exhaling, your abdomen and chest push outward instead of inward. Many women have been conditioned to this style of breathing due to the "suck it in" cultural standards, corsets, and so on. Reverse breathing is not a natural way of breathing. It is a style of breathing known to be used in yoga and qigong, but it is important to understand that there is an intention and purpose behind it.

To find out if you are a chest breather or reverse breather, simply lie down on your back and place your hand on your abdomen. When you inhale, notice if our hand rises up toward the ceiling or pulls in further in toward your back and when you exhale notice if your abdomen draws in or pushes out. If when inhaling, your abdomen pulls in and if when exhaling your abdomen pushes out, you are reverse breathing.

By learning to breathe more effectively, it can do wonders for your health.

## Water

Clean water in our body is just as important as clean water outside our body. Two-thirds of the human body is made of up of water and two-thirds of this water is inside the trillions of cells in the body. Dehydration is much more common than most people suspect. Throughout our evolutionary history, eating and drinking went hand in hand as most foods were high water content foods. Our body's signals for hunger and thirst are very closely related and are often confused. In the animal kingdom, all foods are high water content foods and naturally contain the minerals needed for proper hydration on a cellular level. For humans this is very different. Nowadays much of our food is dehydrated and devoid of hydrating minerals, partly for ease of storage and transport.

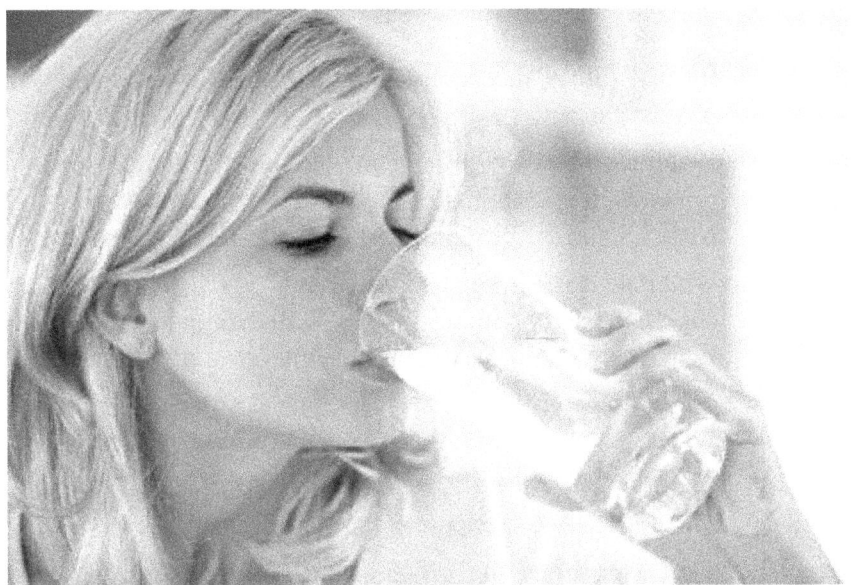

Dehydration is easily misdiagnosed and many people are unaware that their body is thirsting for water. Dehydration is known to cause a variety of health problems and conditions. In "You're Not Sick You're Thirsty" by F Batmanghelidj M.D., he gives a list of 46 Reasons To Drink More Water:

- Without water, nothing lives. Without quality water, nothing thrives.
- Dehydration first suppresses and eventually kills some aspects of the body.
- Water is the main source of energy – it is the "cash flow" of the body.
- Water generates electrical and magnetic energy inside each and every cell of the body – it provides the power to live.
- Water is the bonding adhesive in the architectural design of the cell structure.

- Water prevents DNA damage and makes its repair mechanisms more efficient – less abnormal DNA is made.
- Water increases greatly the efficiency of the immune system in the bone marrow, where the immune system is formed (all is mechanisms) – including its efficiency against cancer.
- Water is the main solvent for all foods, vitamins and minerals. It is used in the breakdown of food into smaller particles and their eventual metabolism and assimilation.
- Water energizes food, and food particles are then able to supply the body with this energy during digestion. This is why food without water has absolutely no energy value for the body.
- Water increases the body's rate of absorption of essential substances in food.
- Water is used to transport all substances inside the body.
- Water increases the efficiency of red blood cells in collecting oxygen in the lungs.
- When water reaches a cell, it brings the cell oxygen and takes the waste gases to the lungs for disposal.
- Water clears toxic waste from different parts of the body and takes it to the liver and kidneys for disposal.
- Water is the main lubricant in the joint spaces and helps prevents arthritis and back pain.
- Water is used in the spinal discs to make them "shock absorbing water cushions".
- Water is the best lubricating laxative and prevents constipation.
- Water helps reduce the risk of heart attacks and strokes.
- Water prevents clogging of arteries in the heart and the brain.
- Water is essential for the body's cooling (sweat) and heating (electrical) systems.

- Water gives us power and electrical energy for all brain functions, most particularly thinking.
- Water is directly needed for the efficient manufacture of all neurotransmitters, including serotonin.
- Water is directly needed for the production of all hormones made by the brain, including melatonin.
- Water can help prevent attention deficit disorder in children and adults.
- Water increases efficiency at work; it expands your attention span.
- Water is a better pick-me-up than any other beverage in the world and it has no side effects.
- Water helps reduce stress, anxiety and depression.
- Water restores normal sleep rhythms.
- Water helps reduce fatigue – it gives us the energy of youth.
- Water makes the skin smoother and helps decrease the effects of aging.
- Water gives luster and shine to the eyes.
- Water helps prevent glaucoma.
- Water normalizes the blood-manufacturing systems in the bone marrow – it helps prevent leukemia and lymphoma.
- Water is absolutely vital for making the immune system more efficient in different regions to fight infections and cancer cells where they are formed.
- Water dilutes the blood and prevents it from clotting during circulation.
- Water decreases premenstrual pains and hot flashes.
- Water and heartbeats create the dilution and waves that keep things from sedimenting in the blood stream.
- The human body has no stored water to draw on during dehydration. This is why you must drink regularly and throughout the day.

- Dehydration prevents sex hormone production – one of the primary causes of impotence and loss of libido.
- Drinking water separates the sensations of thirst and hunger.
- To lose weight, water is the best way to go – drink water on time and lose weight without much dieting. Also, you will not eat excessively when you feel hungry but are in fact only thirsty for water.
- Dehydration causes deposits of toxic sediments in the tissue spaces, joints, kidneys, liver, brain and skin. Water will clear these deposits.
- Water reduces the incidence of morning sickness in pregnancy.
- Water integrates mind and body functions. It increases ability to realize goals and purpose.
- Water prevents the loss of memory as we age. It helps reduce the risk of Alzheimer's disease, multiple sclerosis, Parkinson's disease and Lou Gehrig's disease.
- Water helps reverse addictive urges, including those for caffeine, alcohol and some drugs.

As a result, we can see how it is of utmost importance not only to ensure we are giving our bodies enough water, but also that the quality of water we are putting into our bodies is the purest. For that very reason, it is necessary to know our water source, the possible contaminants contained in our water, and support movements that will help to keep our water clean.

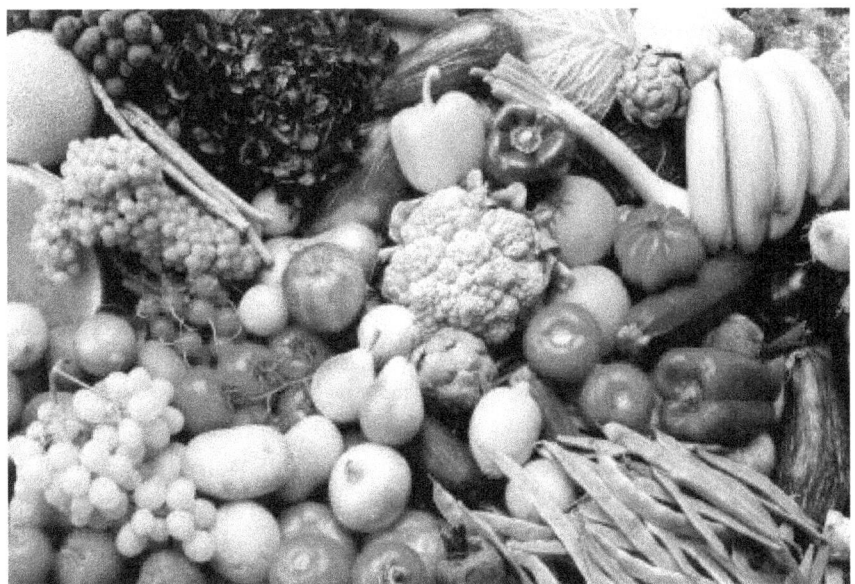

## Food

"The food you eat can be either the safest and most powerful form of medicine or the slowest form of poison". — Ann Wigmore

Eating is essentially the process of internalizing your external environment. One could say you are literally merging with your environment. The kind of food we eat and the quality of food (micro environments) that we allow into our body can lead us on a path toward health or imbalance.

In the same way we take responsibility for the quality of water we put into our bodies, it is important that we do the same with our food. In fact, as we move up the food chain, the pollutants in our water and environment become more concentrated in the organisms we eat, especially animals.

Pesticides are responsible for many serious health issues and environmental problems.

The Environmental Working Group estimates that every day, 1.1 million children eat food that, even after it is washed, contains an unsafe dose of 13 organophosphate pesticides. Of those children, 106,600 ate food that exceeds the EPA's own safe daily dosage level for adults by 10 times or more. The EWG offers a Shopper's Guide to Pesticides in Produce™ available at ewg.org/foodnews/

The purest form of food, which is what I consider healthy food, comes from organic, non-gmo, and locally grown sources that have had the least amount of processing. To ensure you are eating the best quality and least processed food, get into the habit of reading labels and questioning where your food comes from.

Think of food like your own body. Is the food you're about to ingest natural, alive, vibrant, and fresh or has it been manufactured, treated with toxic pesticides, or synthetically enhanced? Does it come from a healthy stress free animal, or one that is sick and fighting infections? Is it a food we have evolved to eat over for a few million years, a few thousand, a few hundred, or in a lab in the past few months?

There has been much concern over hormone disrupting foods, and hormones added to milk and cattle, but it is often overlooked that these animals themselves contain natural growth hormones and growth factors which are also very potent and have powerful effects on the body, dairy being one example.

The biggest hormone disrupter of all appears to be that of insulin itself. High levels of insulin are toxic to our body, causing increased triglyceride production and weight gain, and much more. When too much insulin is swimming around the body it competes with hormones and nutrients of all sorts for entry into our cells. While insulin has been our best friend for millions of years, in the last couple generations it has started to become our biggest enemy. Of course when one begins to understand its role in the body it can again become a beautiful tool to nourish and strengthen the body. Thanks to little known pioneers in insulin research such as Ron Rosedale, insulin is starting to be understood by the layman and by a select few in the medical field who are waking up to the powerful role insulin plays in the obesity and disease epidemics facing this nation and many others.

Soft drink consumption is linked to overweight and obesity. The risk of obesity is even higher among people who drink diet soda. The findings come from eight years of data collected by Sharon P. Fowler, MPH, and colleagues at the University of Texas Health Science Center, San Antonio. "There was a 41 percent increase in risk of being overweight for every can or bottle of diet soft drink a person consumes each day," Fowler says.

The use of and the amount of alcohol one consumes should also be reconsidered. According to Dr Daniel Amen, a brain health expert, best-selling author and two-time board certified psychiatrist, *"Any amount of alcohol can decrease brain size. I like to say when it comes to the brain, size matters. People who drink alcohol — even the moderate amounts that help prevent heart disease — have a smaller brain volume than those who do not, according to a study in the Archives of Neurology."*

There is a famous saying, "you are what you eat" which can been traced back as early as 1826 in *Physiologie du Gout, ou Meditations de Gastronomie Transcendante* by Anthelme Brillat-Savarin where he wrote, "Tell me what you eat and I will tell you what you are." By applying this thought to our daily nutrition, it can be easy to understand the kinds of foods that make us strong and resilient, and the kind of foods that make us weak.

The major challenge underlying all of this is our culture, and underlying that is our brain which is hard wired to follow the culture/herd in lockstep. Our culture has conditioned our minds to consider healthy food as unappetizing, bland or boring. For example, when people think of introducing healthy food into their lifestyle, celery and carrot sticks come to mind, or green veggie juices, or tofu. Foods like ice cream, chips, and cookies are considered to be "treats" or "goodies", a psychologically pleasing concept. In addition, our pallets are hijacked by highly visual marketing equating junk food with fun and celebration. Our bodies have to further battle a barrage of flavor enhanced foods containing the perfect balance of excessive sugar, salt, spices, acids, biochemically addictive additives, and scent engineering that easily overpowers our capacity to taste and enjoy a variety of natural foods.

The good news is that there is a world of healthy foods out there that taste amazing and we have the power and potential to re-condition and reshape the kind of foods and cravings our bodies have been accustomed to.

As previously mentioned with water, it is necessary to not only know our food source, quality and its effects on our body, but in addition support local farmers, movements, people, and organizations that are committed to keeping our food as clean and green as possible.

## Sunshine

Over the years I have witnessed an increasing amount of concern over sun exposure due to ozone depletion, global warming, and skin cancer along with an increase in sunscreen usage and warnings to deal with this concern. Likewise in the last few years, there has been a huge increase in the studies showing the health benefits of sunshine. Sun exposure has now been shown to prevent literally dozens of major illnesses including cancer. There is no question that too much of anything, even something that is essential and good for you, can become a problem. Clearly one can overdose on vitamins, herbs, drugs, and even water. Too much of just about anything can become toxic in the body. It's the same with our good friend the sun. Sunshine has tremendous health benefits and many scientists have been finding through their research that exposure to sunshine as little as 15 minutes a day 3 times per week has been shown to ward of all sorts of illness and disease, and greatly affect the mood and those battling depression. Sunshine also regulates and balances hormone levels and circadian rhythms so those with sleep issues can also benefit from more sun exposure.

According to a study discussed in Scientific American, "Vitamin D deficiency soars in the U.S.", as three-quarters of U.S. teens and adults are now deficient in vitamin D, the so-called "sunshine vitamin". Vitamin D deficits are increasingly blamed for everything from cancer and heart disease to diabetes, according to new research.

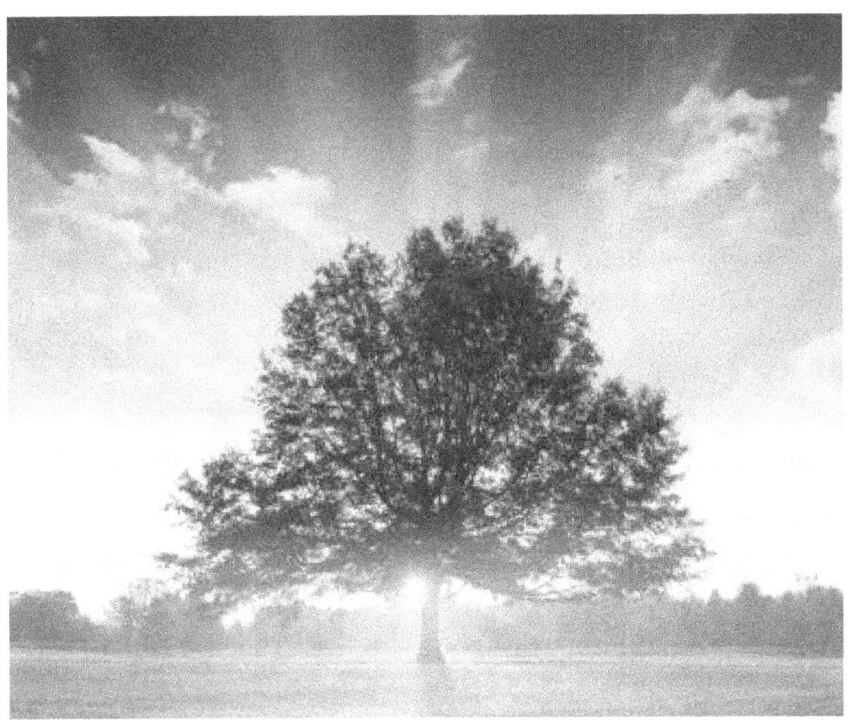

What's also important to understand is that the kind of Vitamin D that sunshine provides is not of the same substance that can be found in a supplement. The so called 'Vitamin D' produced when sun hits the skin, is actually a hormone, not a vitamin. The sunshine hormone has been shown to boost the absorption of nearly every vitamin and mineral that enters the body. The other side of this is that studies have also show that the cells in the eyes properly divide only in the presence of sunlight. Other research has shown the role of sunlight on the pineal gland and its cascading effects in the glandular system of the body, including its strong effects on the hypothalamus which some people consider the master gland.

The problem with this being widely recognized is that there is a whole industry of sun tan lotions, sun protectant cosmetics, sunglasses, and dermatologists warning people left and right about sun damage. With that said, the amount of sunshine needed and what is excessive or considered dangerous will vary from person to person and is related to a number of factors including: genetics, medical history, culture, geography, the time of day, skin color, the season, whether they just showered and used soaps which wash off the body's natural oils/protectants, the amount of time spent in the sun previously, and much more.

Another irony in all of this is that recent research has shown Vitamin D to be perhaps the most important nutrient of all in preventing skin cancer, yet somehow the sun has been blamed for nearly all skin cancers. An interesting fact: There is no hard evidence that regular, moderate sun exposure causes melanomas, for example.

According to an article *Does Sunshine Actually Decrease Dangerous Melanoma Skin Cancers?* By Dr. Mercola on April 28 2012:

*Sensible Sunlight is Protective Against Melanoma. Exposure to sunlight, particularly UVB, is protective against melanoma — or rather, the vitamin D your body produces in response to UVB radiation is protective. As written in The Lancet:*

*"Paradoxically, outdoor workers have a decreased risk of melanoma compared with indoor workers, suggesting that chronic sunlight exposure can have a protective effect."*

*A study in Medical Hypotheses suggested that indoor workers may have increased rates of melanoma because they're exposed to sunlight through windows, and only UVA light, unlike UVB, can pass through window glass. At the same time, these indoor workers, who get three to nine times less solar UV exposure than outdoor workers, are missing out on exposure to the beneficial UVB rays, and have lower levels of vitamin D. The study even noted that indoor UV actually breaks down vitamin D3 formed after outdoor UVB exposure, which would therefore make vitamin D3 deficiency and melanoma risk even worse.*

Some people might argue against all this, citing data showing that skin cancer is on the rise, yet this overlooks the fact that *all* cancers are on the rise.

According to an article *Obesity-Linked Cancers Increased* in The Wall Street Journal on March 28 2012:

*Several cancers linked to obesity and a sedentary lifestyle rose every year from 1999 through 2008, even as improved screening and a sharp decline in the number of smokers have helped push down the rate of new cancer diagnoses overall across the U.S., according to a report released Wednesday.*

*Rates of cancers of the kidney, pancreas, lower esophagus and uterus increased annually through 2008, the latest data available, according to the Annual Report to the Nation on the Status of Cancer. Rates of breast cancer in women at least 50 years old declined 1.3% annually from 1999 to 2005 but rose slightly between 2005 and 2008.*

According to the National Cancer Institute the top three most common cancers in 2012 are:
- Prostate
- Breast
- Lung

### Exercise/Movement

Our bodies have been naturally designed to move. Movement is linked to every function and process in the body. One of the biggest problems in today's modern day culture is that our society has adapted to a lifestyle that encourages little to no movement. This is referred to as being 'sedentary', which literally means 'to sit'. Interestingly enough a sedentary lifestyle can not only lead to obesity, disease, and chiropractic issues, but it can also easily be shown how it indirectly leads to an unsustainable economy and environment and life for all. Here are some examples of how to transition out of a sedentary lifestyle:
- riding a bike or walking versus using a car
- making or growing your own food vs. eating out
- rather than watching sports and dancing and nature tours on TV vs. one can actually participate in the activity
- Finding ways to begin earning one's livelihood through farming, gardening, nature tours, building, caretaking, landscaping, eco-tourism, etc, instead of sitting 8-10 hours behind a corporate desk.
- using a standup workstation versus a sit-down desk

By adding more movement in our lives, we will contribute to improving the quality of our health, and we will also create less pollution and naturally head down the road toward a truly sustainable lifestyle.

Exercise has so many physical and mental benefits. Here are a few:
- Reduces insulin resistance
- Increases bone density
- Improves cardiovascular and respiratory health
- Regulates the production of stress hormones
- Promotes neuronal growth in the brain
- Stimulates learning centers of the brain
- Increases energy levels

**Below are a couple of quotes about movement taken from the film The Cure Is U: Cureisu.com**

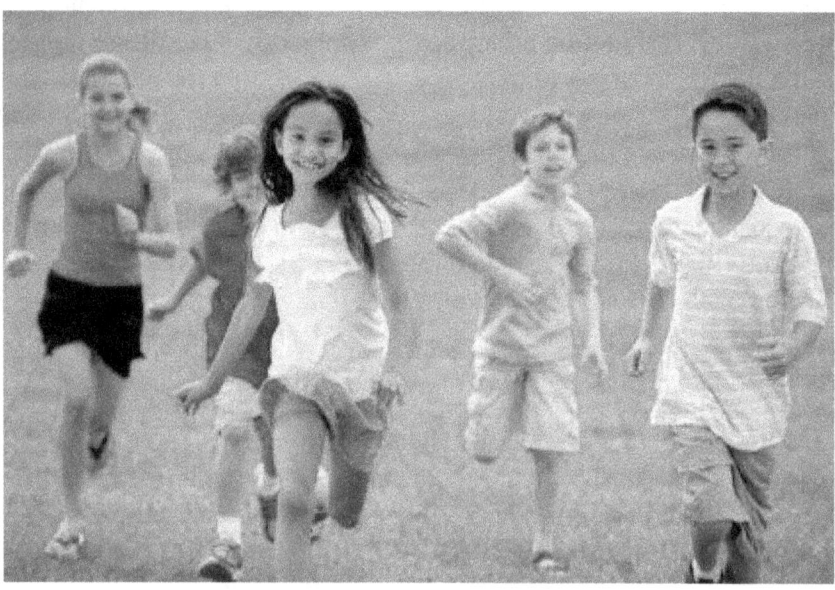

"Human beings are moving approximately 90% less than they did forty years ago, yet we maintain the same biology, the same genes, and the same requirements that human beings had throughout their evolution. If we do not get enough adequate movement, we do not pump the body, clean the body, and therefore we cannot maintain vitality" ~ Paul Chek, founder of The Chek Institute

"We usually exercise for every reason from the neck down, but in reality when you do exercise, what it ends up doing is affecting everything from the neck up. When you move physically your brain chemistry changes and when your brain chemistry changes, there is a greater likelihood that you'll succeed when it comes to finding things in your life that bring you happiness and joy that also create productivity in your life."~ Tony Horton, Leading Expert in Exercise, Health and Wellbeing

## Emotions/Thoughts

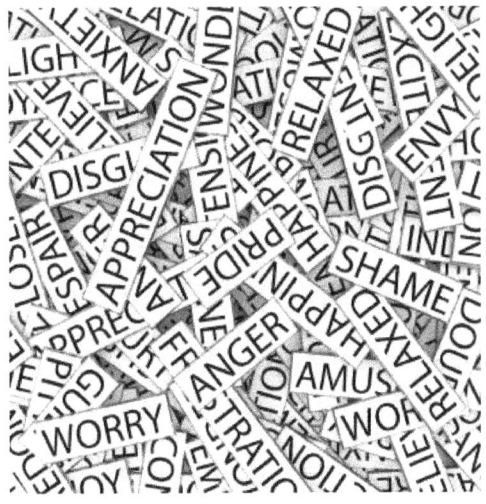

Although the body and mind are usually studied or looked at as two separate components, they work closely in conjunction with another and can ultimately be considered as one. Thoughts and emotions are intricately tied to the various functions of our body and can support or challenge our body's health.

Brain health and its connection to our moods, relationships, and our cognitive function have been brought to the forefront by speakers like Dr Daniel Amen M.D., who wrote the book "Change Your Brian, Change Your Life". He has studied many thousands of brain scans and many of the patterns he sees in his practice are clear as pertaining to dark areas on the brains scans caused by drug use, alcohol abuse, sports injuries, head trauma, toxic work environment, nutritional deficiencies, and other factors that damage the brain and cause poor brain health and create poor brain circulation. Each type of brain injury leaves a very specific fingerprint upon the brain.

Poor brain health can lead to mood and behavioral disorders and can greatly affect relationships and produce negative thinking patterns which can then lead to further destructive habits which can then damage the brain even further. It becomes a downward spiral that can be easily cured through proper brain nutrition.

Other researchers and scientists take the approach that disease and illness can be tied directly to an emotion that has been unreleased within us, or a trauma that has set off a defense mechanism within the body. When we are born, we have a natural tendency to release and process our emotions. It is natural part of our human function, but as we grow, most of us become conditioned to suppress or ignore our emotions. When we suppress or ignore our emotions, we diminish our vitality and risk exposing ourselves to a variety of acute and chronic health issues. Our posture changes, our breath becomes shallower, and our energy levels are affected. In addition our thoughts change and become very negative and self-destructive, so much so that they can signal the body to react in a variety of negative ways. Most of us are unaware of our thoughts and the amount of thoughts that pass through us on a daily basis due to our fast paced lifestyles.

One German physician by the name of Dr. Hamer, has thoroughly documented the effect of shocks on the body in his studies. His studies have been peer reviewed and supported more than 30 times by other doctors and researchers. Dr. Hamer suggests that "nothing in Nature is "diseased" but always biologically meaningful. According to the Five Biological Laws, diseases are not malignancies, as proposed by conventional medicine, but instead are age-old "Biological Special Programs of Nature" that assist an individual during unexpected emotional distress.

Dr. Hamer also suggests that most disease and cancers can be traced back to "unexpected, highly acute, and isolating conflict shocks that occur simultaneously in the PSYCHE, the BRAIN, and on the corresponding ORGAN."

There are many great scientists like those above that you can research, and for those who prefer a movie format, "The Cure Is U" is a documentary film that explains how we can directly influence our state of well-being just by how we think and feel.

## About The Cure Is U

The Cure is U explores the relationship of our emotions to our health and clearly demonstrates how our thoughts not only contribute to disease but may be the most powerful factor in determining whether we succumb to illness and even life threatening disease. So powerful are our thoughts that they can even negate the benefits of even the healthiest of diets. Most experts universally agree that eating a healthy diet and exercising often are key components to our longevity and wellbeing. Now, experts are focusing on a new health paradigm that is shattering the way we look at our health. Doctors, scientists, researchers and health experts are now recognizing that our thinking may be one of the most significant aspects to our overall wellbeing. We now know that our body releases chemicals that either support our health or healing or can destroy it, all based upon what we think and feel. Experts are examining how our thoughts communicate with our heart then to our brain which releases chemicals that either keeps us in health or breaks down our immune system and allows for disease. This profound finding has brought forth a new relationship — that how we feel, our emotions, may be the most overlooked aspect to our health.
www.cureisu.com

## Sleep/Restoration

"Sleep is the best meditation." ~Dalai Lama

Just like air, water, and food, sleep is a vital necessity for life. Sleep assists our body in rejuvenating and restoring what is lost when we are awake, improves memory and learning, controls inflammations, reduces stress, promotes healthy weight, conserves energy, aids in brain function, promotes muscle building and repair, and much more.

Millions of Americans are affected by sleep disorders. According to the Center for Disease Control and Prevention, an estimated 50-70 million US adults have sleep or wakefulness disorder. Persons experiencing sleep insufficiency are also more likely to suffer from chronic diseases such as hypertension, diabetes, depression, and obesity, as well as from cancer, increased mortality, and reduced quality of life and productivity.

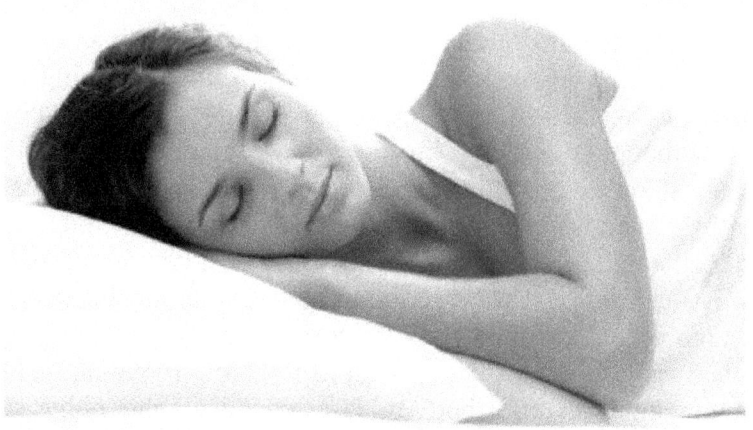

Sleep Deprivation can contribute to the following:

- Depression
- Irritability
- Poor Performance
- Decrease in Productivity
- Mental Fogginess
- Headaches
- Psychosis
- Pain Sensitivity
- Slows Reflexes
- Tremors
- Poor Digestion
- Obesity

- Diabetes
- Unhealthy Behaviors
- Accidents
- Weakened Immune System

To deal with sleep deprivation many have turned to the use of sleep medications.

Prescriptions for sleeping medications topped 56 million in 2008 — a record, according to the research firm IMS Health, up 54% from 2004.

Researchers at Scripps Health, a nonprofit health system in San Diego, estimate that in 2010, sleeping pill use may have contributed to up to 500,000 "excess deaths" in the United States.

Why are so many adults and children affected by sleep disorders? And is the immediate solution to rely on medication?

In order to answer this question, it helps to understand all the components involved in encouraging or preventing a good night's sleep.

- Nutrition (What and how you eat throughout the day and night)
- Sunlight Exposure (Sunshine sets your biological clock. Lack of sunshine inhibits sleep)
- Room Temperature
- Room Environment
- Bed Environment
- Dark Environment
- Sound
- Sleep Routine/Schedule
- Circadian Rhythm (Sleeping between the hours of 10pm and 6am)
- EMF exposure
- Toxic Exposure from products, walls, bedding, carpet, etc.

- Indoor Air Quality
- Exposure late at night to Bright lights, TVs and Computers
- Stress
- Lack of support
- Travel

While all of the above components have a cumulative effect on sleep quality, one of the most overlooked components is that of foods and drinks. Culprits such as caffeine from coffee and theobromine from chocolate, as well as alcohol, adversely affect sleep quality, even with moderate use. These toxins should be avoided as much as possible. Caffeine stays in the body for approximately 24 hours, and even a small amount of alcohol in the evening can prevent deep sleep.

In addition, evaluating the indoor air quality in your bedroom where you may spend an average of six hours or more every night is essential for your well-being. Indoor air quality may be affected by carpeting, fragrances, poor ventilation, bedding, new carpet, new furniture, paint, electronics, pet dander, VOC's, mold, formaldehyde, etc.

Home Air Check is a company that tests your air for these chemicals so that you can identify these household pollutants and do something about it for cleaner, healthier air. For more information, visit their website at homeaircheck.com.

Sleep is essential to reconstruct lost body-protein and to decompose and remove wastes from the body." If you want a green body, a waste free body, then sleep is of utmost importance. Assessing your current lifestyle by evaluating the above components and making a few small changes can encourage and promote a good night's sleep.

## Stress Management

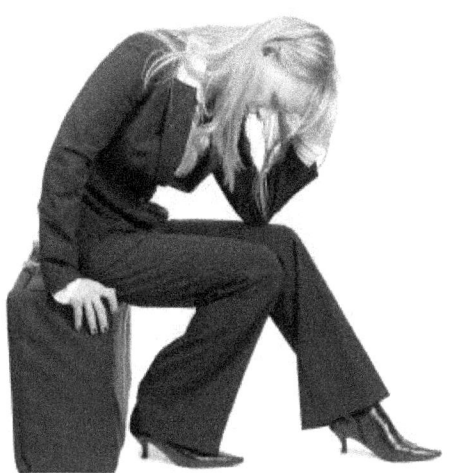

The term "stress", as it is currently used was coined by Hans Selye in 1936, who defined it as "the non-specific response of the body to any demand for change". Changes in one's life may include winning the lottery, getting promoted, getting married, etc....or challenging events like getting a divorce, losing a job, or going bankrupt. There is good stress and bad stress. What it boils down to is how you manage stress.

Stress is more than just your emotional health. While emotional stress can certainly lead to elevated stress levels in the body and no doubt requires healthy management and therapy to get it in balance, there are other causes of excessive stress hormones swimming in your body as well. The major one being the aforementioned: Insulin.

There is no doubt that excessive stress hormones swimming around inside the body are toxic. Many would suggest that they are equally as toxic, if not more so, than the outer chemicals we are warned to avoid.

Many people in the green movement with good reason, are worried about the amounts of chemicals or toxins in their environment; however the body can easily swim with toxins produced by its' own organs in response to sugar. Too much of anything can be toxic, and carbohydrates are no exception.

Diet alone can engulf your body in a torrent of stress hormones, which in excess become toxic, wreaking havoc on your arteries and your entire body, disrupting your hormones, and preventing the uptake of nutrients into your body.

To handle stress some people also resort to the use of drugs, one most commonly thought to be harmless, marijuana.

Cannabis (Marijuana) use should be reconsidered. It is estimated that 15 million Americans use cannabis in a given month—3.4 million are daily users with a duration of 12 months or more, and that every year 2.1 million start using the drug. According to the Council on Alcoholism, *smoking marijuana causes decreased activity in the posterior temporal lobes of the brain. Cannabis narrows and squeezes down blood flow, leading to brain cell damage and cell death. Dr Daniel Amen's research has found that it particularly affects the temporal lobes. This damage creates greatly enlarged black spots on brain scans that are easily seen. This happens primarily in the area of the brain responsible for memory. "Dr. Amen suggests that this is the reason for the poor memory and lack of motivation that chronic users often report."*

According to the American Institute of Stress;

*There are numerous emotional and physical disorders that have been linked to stress including depression, anxiety, heart attacks, stroke, hypertension, immune system disturbances that increase susceptibility to infections, a host of viral linked disorders ranging from the common cold and herpes to AIDS and certain cancers, as well as autoimmune diseases like rheumatoid arthritis and multiple sclerosis. In addition stress can have direct effects on the skin (rashes, hives, atopic dermatitis, the gastrointestinal system (GERD, peptic ulcer, irritable bowel syndrome, ulcerative colitis) and can contribute to insomnia and degenerative neurological disorders like Parkinson's disease. In fact, it's hard to think of any disease in which stress cannot play an aggravating role or any part of the body that is not affected.*

Learning to manage our stress is essential. Having a well-balanced diet helps to control and manage stress. When your diet is in balance, managing your stress, establishing healthy habits, boundaries and creating a lifestyle that promotes emotional well-being and balance becomes a lot easier. There are also a number of stress management techniques, resources, and even stress management coaches that can offer help.

## Energy

The study of energy is quite fascinating. Most of us relate energy to our outer environment in the form of electricity. We also have inner energy that contributes to our main source of power. In Chinese Medicine, energy is considered one's chi or life force.

The human body's main power comes from the mitochondrion. It is believed to be *our* source of energy. Our main sources of energy come from:

- Adenosine triphosphate (ATP)
- Oxygen
- Glucose
- Fats and Amino Acids

So how do we make the body more efficient, and thus more green?

- Deep sleep creates a clean and efficiently running waste-free body.
- Breathing efficiently through diaphragmatic breathing.
- Staying hydrated.
- CRAN-Calorie Restriction with Adequate Nutrition means that we eat nutrient dense foods so that we aren't taking in unnecessary calories to meet nutrient requirements (and cravings) in the body. When the body gets what it needs, the appetite diminishes. CRAN research on animals has shown that various species of animals can live anywhere between thirty and two-hundred percent longer. They have studied several dozen species, including primates, and the results are uniform throughout.

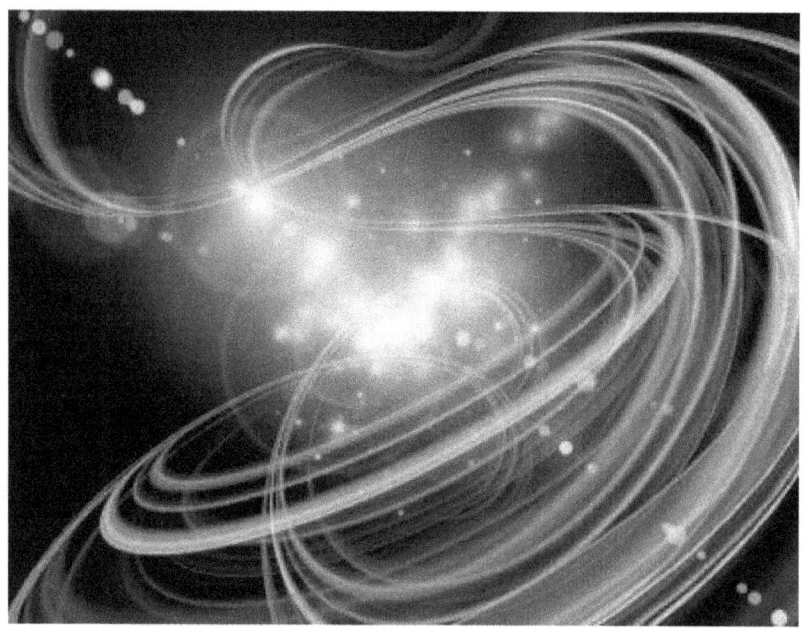

- Keep your body insulin sensitive. High insulin levels lead to insulin resistance which leads to essentially sugar resistance which keeps adequate sugar from entering the cell. When your body becomes insulin resistant, it also becomes nutrient resistant as the entry of nutrients into the cells becomes less and less fluid. The body then tries to consume more of everything as it starts to starve on a cellular level. This leads to fatigue and a host of illnesses which then makes one heavily dependent upon medical intervention.
- Prevention is far more efficient than intervention. When illness is prevented, far less resources and money and economic structures are needed. The industry of prevention could easily be one twentieth the size of the current Allopathic model of disease treatment and intervention. All the energy could go toward sustainable living and greening the planet and the body.
- Maintain optimal body weight. When the body is carrying around less weight, it has more energy and becomes a more efficient machine. Overeating means more energy is diverted to digestion, assimilation, and

detoxification of the food stuffs coming in. A huge percentage of your daily energy expenditure goes for these three food related processes.

## Environment

The environment we live in has many affects to our physical and mental well-being. Some of us are more sensitive than others to our environment.

Components in our varied environments include:
- Culture
- Climate
- Nature
- Resources
- Population
- Noise Level
- Air Quality
- Water Quality
- Food Quality

Different environments can stimulate and entertain us, like NYC or Las Vegas. Other environments can calm us and slow our mind down, like a secluded beach or forest.

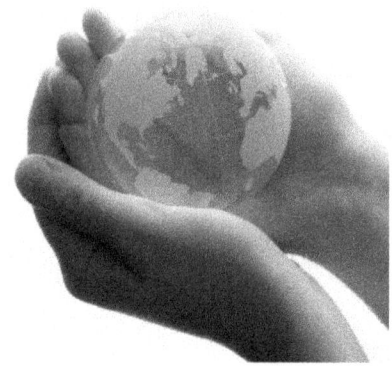

Some climates can create mood imbalances like Seasonal Affective Disorder which lead to other challenges. Other climates with lots of sunshine and UV rays can enhance our mood.

Some local cultures support sustainable living, and others encourage consumerism and environment destruction.

Some cities have very clean air, and some have very dirty air. Some have dirty chemical laden water, and others have natural spring water.

One should seek out an environment that supports one's own goals so that one is not swimming against the current of that particular local.

## Intuition

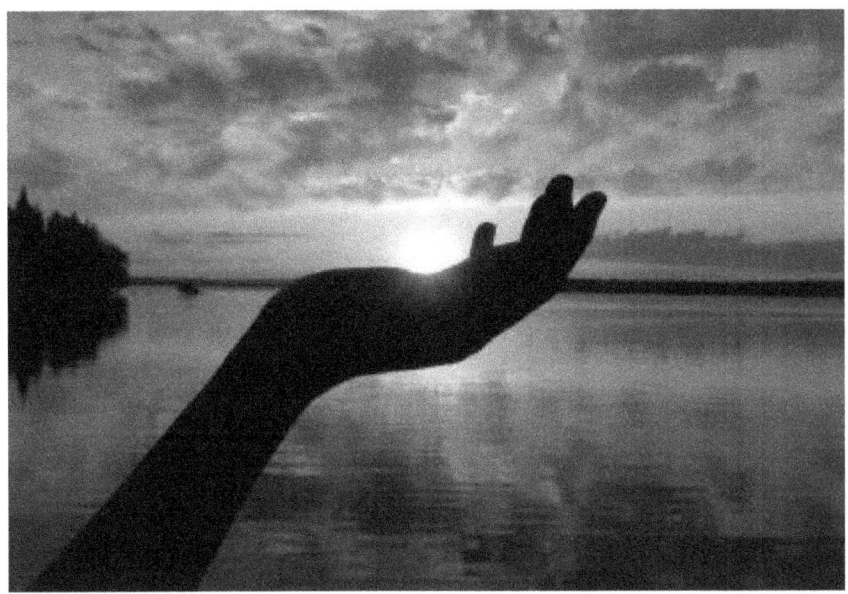

Intuition is a powerful tool. It gives us the ability to understand something clearly without the need for analysis. Florence Scovel, a theologian, once said, "Intuition is the spiritual faculty that doesn't explain; it seemingly points the way."

All of us are born with an innate ability to use our intuition but overtime analytic reasoning usually becomes our main source of reliance. As Krishnamurti once said "Analysis is paralysis". The thinking mind has become so analytical, due to our perceived fragmentation of that which is a whole. When one sees life in fragments, one is always analyzing and thinking about how to relate to the various fragments and how all the fragments fit together. When one discovers that life is one seamless whole, one can relax and feel one's way through life, guided by the intuition of the body, feeling what feels right and healthy, and moving away from that which doesn't feel nurturing. One doesn't get paralyzed in analysis and decision making, rather one can intuit from feeling the whole of Life, the entire universe, and act from that place of intuition.

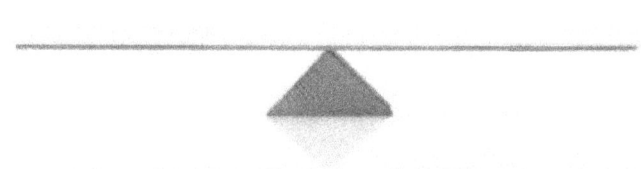

## Balance

Air, water, food, sunshine, exercise/movement, emotions/thoughts, sleep/restoration, stress management, energy, environment, and intuition are all vital components to achieving balance and well-being.

We all go through various fluctuations and stages in our life where one or more of these components may need more attention than some others. One is not more important than the other, though certainly some can have more powerful effects upon your body than others.

Once you are able to see and feel all these components, you can begin to put them all in their natural place of balance. It is very easy to give one component of health all the importance, or create a cure all or panacea for all diseases.

All the components covered in this chapter play essential and seamless roles in the bigger picture of sustainability which includes our personal lives and all of humanity on our planet and in our Universe.

# *Preconception*

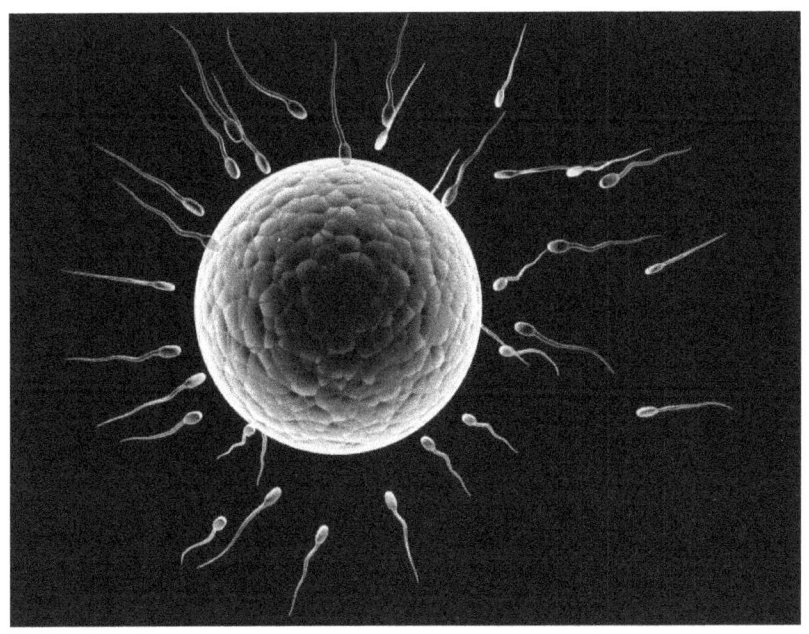

As some of you may have discovered, conception often comes when you least expect it. In a world in which drinking and drugs use (both prescription and recreational) is so prevalent, it is very common for mothers to find themselves in a situation where they have discovered they are already a month or two along in their pregnancy, but they have still been taking drugs or drinking heavily on the weekends, not sleeping enough, or they may find themselves worried about how all their recent stress may have affected the baby that they didn't even know was there. This is all too common and all the more reason to commit oneself to a healthy and green lifestyle.

For some couples the problem is a very different one: Infertility.

According to the Centers for Disease Control the number of women aged 25 and younger who are struggling with infertility, has increased by 50% in the last decade and that figure is rising!

About forty percent of infertility cases come from the male.

When being diagnosed with infertility it is usually unexpected and can leave one feeling at a loss, disappointed, powerless, frustrated, guilty, worthless, and a failure.

It takes time to process the news and then gather the information necessary to sort it all out. The future is suddenly uncertain and one's hopes and dreams can suddenly feel as if they are slipping away. During this time it is important to seek support whether it is from family, friends, or a group, as it can be very easy to place the blame on oneself or one another.

Many times one reacts quickly to the uncomfortable emotions and suddenly begins to fight against the news. One can make rash decisions that may not be the most suitable or logical.

It is important to take the space and time to not only deal with your emotions but also look deeper into what is happening in your body and your surroundings. This can become an opportunity to learn how to take care of your body and boost your own vitality and fertility. The body is normally designed to reproduce and infertility is an opportunity to question your overall health, or that of your partner, your environment, and take steps together to heal and nourish one another back to a state of vitality, especially in cases where infertility has been determined to come from a medical issue.

## Evaluating Infertility

As difficult and challenging facing infertility may be, I believe our bodies are giving us a tremendous opportunity when we are faced with this challenge. Our body has its' own natural intelligence and infertility is our body's way of protecting us and the potential of creating another human life in an unsustainable environment. It's our body's way of alerting us that our body's reproductive and/or immune systems have been compromised whether this has been due to poor lifestyle habits, toxic environmental exposures, or medical issues.

There are many options when dealing with infertility and the most important thing is to know your options so you can make informed decisions along the way. It is a time to evaluate the possible imbalances in your lifestyle, exposure to toxins, or medical issues that may be attributing to infertility. The cause of infertility is probably not related to just one factor but a number of factors.

Let's take a look at the areas that can affect fertility in men and women:

- Age
- Stress
- Sleep Deprivation
- Poor Nutrition
- Athletic Training
- Medications
- Medical Issues
- Overweight or Underweight
- Smoking
- Alcohol Use
- Home and Work Environment
- Hormone Disruptors found in Products ingested through the mouth, inhaled, or absorbed through the skin

In the article at The Puristat Digestive Wellness Center (Puristat.com), *Discovering the Link Between Infertility and*

*Detoxification*, Dr Jesse Hanley, MD and Jo Jordan wrote the following (The remainder of this article is featured at the end of this chapter.):

"French scientists discovered a connection between infertility and environmental toxins in the 1850s. In addition to an unusually high rate of miscarriage, they noticed that lead workers' wives had trouble conceiving. Their discovery was hardly groundbreaking; the Romans had already made the connection between infertility and environmental toxins in the second century!"

Dr. Hanley says, "Yes, there are damaging and deadly toxins out there, but cleansing your body makes a world of difference."

A study conducted by the University of Surrey showed that couples with a previous history of infertility who made changes in their lifestyle, diet and took nutritional supplements had an 80 percent success rate. Given that the success rate for assisted conception is around 20 percent, it's worth considering lifestyle changes first.

According to The World Health Organization, they estimate that we could prevent more than 80 percent of all chronic illnesses by improving our lifestyles in simple ways, like working to reduce our exposure to environmental pollutants and eating a healthier diet.

Even when it comes to sex, you can go green to boost your fertility! For example, sex products such as oils, lubricants, and toys are commonly known to contain irritants and hormone disruptors. Select products that are non-toxic.

Most people who seek to treat their infertility are first referred to medical treatment. I am not suggesting it should not be a possible consideration; it absolutely should, but I believe this is a route one should take when it is determined that the cause of infertility is not coming from one's lifestyle or environment. Additionally, when I speak with women and couples who were first referred to medical treatment, upon learning there were other options to take into consideration, they inform me that if they had known all their options, they would most likely have not started with medical treatment.

Medical treatments may include:
- Fertility drugs
- Surgery

- Artificial insemination
- In vitro fertilization (IVF)
- Gamete intrafallopian transfer (GIFT)
- Zygote intrafallopian transfer (ZIFT)
- Intracytoplasmic sperm injection (ICSI)
- Donor eggs and embryos
- Gestational carriers (also known as surrogate mothers)

Natural Treatments can include:
- Homeopathy
- Acupuncture
- Chinese Medicine
- Nutrition
- Yoga
- Meditation
- Stress Management
- Eliminating Environmental Toxic Exposures

Before making a decision about how to treat your infertility, it may be very helpful to perform your own lifestyle and environmental assessment looking at the various areas that can affect fertility as we covered above. Evaluate each component and ask yourself on a scale of 1-10 how well you are managing each (1 being the least managed and 10 being the most managed). This will at least provide you a starting point and a good idea if your lifestyle or environment may be the main cause of your infertility.

## Discovering the Link between Infertility and Detoxification

Source: The Puristat Digestive Wellness Center/Puristat.com
*by Dr. Jesse Hanley, MD and Jo Jordan*

French scientists discovered a connection between infertility and environmental toxins in the 1850s. In addition to an unusually high rate of miscarriage, they noticed that lead workers' wives had trouble conceiving.

Their discovery was hardly groundbreaking; the Romans had already made the connection between infertility and environmental toxins in the second century!

As our environment has become more toxic, infertility rates have skyrocketed, too. In the United States alone, infertility affects over six million American women and men, approximately ten percent of the reproductive-age population, according to the American Society for Reproductive Medicine.[1]

Infertility is now such a critical health problem that in 2006, New Jersey Congressman Frank Pallone Jr. unveiled his plan to set up infertility task force legislation. The group called for more research related to environmental toxins, citing specific examples of increased infertility in patients exposed to contaminated water.[2]

## Research Turns up Alarming Infertility Facts

As more and more people struggle with infertility, research is unearthing startling new data on what, exactly, is at least partly to blame for this near epidemic.

### The Estrogen Effect

Women and men require a proper balance of natural estrogens in order to be successful reproductively. Unfortunately, research suggests that widespread environmental estrogens – chemicals that have the ability to mimic our natural estrogens – are creating infertility havoc by confusing the body's estrogen receptors.

These estrogen mimics – also known as endocrine or hormone disruptors – are found in ordinary, everyday items such as personal care products and toiletries, spermicides, and pesticides. As well, they're a breakdown product of the plastics (polyvinyl chloride, also known as PVC) used in some water jugs and baby bottles.[3]

Other culprits include the antioxidant preservative butylated hydroxyanisole (BHA). A carcinogen, this preservative is found in food and personal care products such as foundations, concealers, and other cosmetics. Even at fairly low doses, it can cause breast cancer cells to multiply.[4]

### Grandmaternal Effects:

"There is no doubt that by continuously ingesting pesticides and other chemicals known to be estrogen mimics, we have created endocrine problems...in other words, a long-term infertility crisis for both men and women, their children, and their children's children, and so on," says Dr. Jesse Hanley.

The effect on fertility of all this toxic activity can be the development of endometriosis, ectopic pregnancy, miscarriage, endometriosis, lactation failure, and infertility in women. For males, estrogen mimicry can result in development without testes, undescended testes, hypospadias (an abnormality of the opening of the penis), abnormally small penises, testicular cancer, or poor semen quality.[5]

And while a mimic may block the action of true estrogen – resulting in a myriad of infertility problems – according to current research, in the worst case scenarios imposters can actually redirect cellular behavior[6] for generations.

In other words, their affects aren't simply limited to the person who has been exposed to these environmental toxins; evidence suggests that the genes of developing fetuses can be permanently reprogrammed by exposure to estrogen mimics, and that this effect can then be passed on for at least three more generations.[7]

The same research points out that in addition to infertility problems, a good portion of test subjects in estrogen mimicry studies also showed signs of kidney disease and tumors.

### Infertility Is Preventable and Treatable

"Yes, there are damaging and deadly toxins out there, but cleansing your body makes a world of difference," says Dr. Hanley. "It really does help to implement twenty-first century solutions for twenty-first century problems."

But the news isn't all bad. After all, if scientific discoveries are changing the way we think about disease development, then we can create a new plan of attack for disease preventives, too!

If we know that disease can be triggered by environmental factors, and carried forward to future generations, then it's important to arm ourselves with the knowledge necessary to avoid whatever known toxics we can.

We know, for example, that twenty to twenty-five percent of miscarriages are related to immune system problems,[8] so it makes sense to focus our health regimens on what's good for the immune system.

Since the late 1970s, we've known that ingesting MSG (monosodium glutamate) greatly reduces the chances of becoming pregnant,[9] so it's vital to avoid processed, junk, and fake foods, which are generally full of additives, preservatives, artificial flavoring and coloring...among other ingredients that can negatively affect your health.

Lifestyle choices are crucial to maximizing fertility. According to Dr. Wolfram Nolten, Endocrinology and Metabolism, University of Wisconsin, "Twenty percent of all cases where the male is the only contributing factor to infertility can be corrected by lifestyle."[10]

## Four Steps toward Protecting Your Fertility

While it is nearly impossible to completely avoid exposure to environmental toxins, it is possible to identify potential fertility hazards in your immediate environment, and create a less toxic environment by stamping them out. Here is what Puristat recommends:

**Step 1:** Help Your Immune System – Lessen the Load with Colon and Liver Cleansings

**Step 2**: Boost Your Immune System – Take a Multi-vitamin

**Step 3**: Eat Right to Keep Fertile – Avoid the Standard American Diet and Other Toxic Traps

**Step 4**: Clean Up – Use Toxic-free Personal Care and Household Products

## Maximizing Fertility

"After thirty years of observing the causes of infertility worldwide, as well as witnessing infertility indicators, I can say with absolute confidence that if you do everything to ensure you are having three bowel movements a day, you will be helping your body become more fertile," says Dr. Hanley.

Know that the lifestyle choices you make within your immediate environment, combined with changes to your health regimen, can go a long way toward protecting yourself and future generations from the trauma of infertility. The sooner you get started, the better your chances will be of overcoming infertility.

## Step 1: Give Your Immune System a Break

"When you detoxify, whether you're male or female, you're more likely to get pregnant, period," says Dr. Hanley. "Cleansings improve elimination, making it easier for your body to get rid of all the bad stuff that has accumulated."

### Lessen the Load with Colon and Liver Cleansings.

Environmental and dietary toxins tax the limits of our bodies' immune systems. With half-a-million chemicals in the environment alone – including the thousands it takes to grow and process our food and the nearly six thousand chemicals and additives in our diet – our bodies must constantly battle to rid themselves of damaging and deadly toxins.

If your body's reserves are constantly being taxed by the energy it takes just to keep excess toxins at bay, then it will be unable to fight off ordinary illnesses. And even a little blip in the immune system can affect fertility. The flu, for example, can slow down a man's sperm production, and any illness that results in a fever can affect both sperm production and quality.

Remember that all the toxins that you ingest, drink, breathe in, and absorb through your skin end up in your liver and gastrointestinal (GI) tract. Here, they wait to be expelled from your colon in the form of waste. The longer they have to wait, more time they have to wreak havoc on your reproductive and other systems.

Colonic irrigation and herbal cleansings can help to remove toxins, parasites, and mucus that have built up in your colon. By flushing out impacted waste, passing stool is easier, and transit times are improved.

Removing impurities also goes a long way toward helping your body absorb nutrients, and enhancing energy levels. Your immune system can get back to the business of providing you with immunity, rather than struggling under the weight of toxic build-up.

Cleansings promote regularity...and more productivity in the bathroom means quicker elimination of environmental toxins from the colon. By creating less opportunity for impurities to be absorbed into the body's reproductive organs, you're taking your fertility out of toxic jeopardy.

A liver cleanse is the next step on the road to a complete purge of toxins, and protecting your reproductive system. Liver cleanses comprised of milk thistle are recommended by some doctors because they're proving to be effective in helping to alleviate the effects of an unhealthy diet, and the burden it places on the immune system...and every other system in the body, including your reproductive system.

Once you become pregnant, Puristat recommends proceeding with caution when using our *Cleanse* as it contains cascara sagrada. This herb is laxative in nature, and ought to be used sparingly, or in combinations with other herbs, during pregnancy. Before continuing a cleanse regimen, consult with your health care provider regarding the benefits and risks of using cascara sagrada during pregnancy.

## Step 2: Boost Your Immune System

### Take a Multi-vitamin.

Eating your veggies is no longer enough to keep our immune systems functioning in peak condition. The soil in which we grow our food is so depleted that it is virtually impossible to get proper sustenance without a supplement...no matter how well you eat.

A rich, superior-grade multi-vitamin / mineral supplement, therefore, is essential to good health and maximizing fertility potential. With a multi-vitamin you can be assured that you're taking the right combination...one that enables vitamins and minerals to work synergistically in your metabolic and enzymatic systems.

Choose a multi-vitamin that contains calcium, magnesium, and essential fatty acids. This will help your body make up for what is lacking in your food, as well as work toward nourishing your cellular functioning – a vital aspect of maximizing fertility.

For men, a daily multi-vitamin can help provide selenium, zinc, and folic acid — these trace nutrients are vital for optimal sperm production and function. A multi-vitamin containing antioxidants such as vitamins C and E, may even help to protect sperm from damage.

## Step 3: Eat Right to Keep Fertile

**Avoid the Standard American Diet and Other Toxic Traps.**

Most people realize that eating a diet heavily based in processed, junk, and fake foods can result in obesity. It's important to know that obesity can also create fertility problems. In addition, there are some nasty truths about much of the food we casually consume that may have a more profound impact on fertility than we might have once believed.

Here are some foods to avoid and some, hopefully, compelling reasons to delete them from the menu:

### Trans fats:

Ingesting margarine – or any of the numerous other fake food products containing trans fats – you are actually incorporating damaged molecules into the cellular structure of your body!

It's hardly surprising, then, that many chronic health conditions – including infertility – have been linked to diets rich in trans fats. Since they are unhealthy, provide no nutritional benefit, and are easy to avoid, why not eliminate trans fats from your diet?

### Processed, junk, and fake foods:

These so-called foods are full of preservatives, antioxidants, artificial coloring and flavoring, additives, sweeteners, and stabilizers...none of which do hopeful moms' or dads' bodies a lick of good. In fact, some of these ingredients are known to interfere with fertility in shocking ways...for generations to come.

In addition, the processes used to produce these products – such as bleaching and refining – deplete any real food that's used of most of its goodness. Processes such as irradiation – the use of x-rays or gamma radiation on food – have had harmful effects on test animals;

they developed increased numbers of cells with chromosome abnormalities, and had unexplained stillbirths.

Worse, food packaging – among other products we use everyday – has been linked to unimaginable consequences.

There is one thing that all these foods, and the effect of the methods used to process them, have in common:

### Energy Output > Exceeds Nutritional Input

In other words, it costs your body a great deal more to digest, absorb, and eliminate them than they offer your body by way of nutritional value – an extremely poor return on your investment that can leave your body sluggish, your immune system depleted, and your chance of remaining healthy and fertile greatly diminished.

## Step 4: Clean Up Your Own Backyard

### Use Toxic-free Personal Care and Household Products.

Every day, we are exposed to toxins in our environment. While to some degree they are simply a fact of twenty-first century living that we can't avoid, there are many things we can do to ensure our home and work places are as toxin-free as possible.

### Personal Care Products.

Know that many ingredients used in cosmetics and personal care products are the same toxic ingredients used in paints, plastics, and pesticides; if you don't recognize an ingredient, find out what it is, and how it can affect your fertility.

In addition to rating an assortment of household products, this guide lists many chemical hazards and their effects: http://www.lesstoxicguide.ca/default.aspx?fetch=personal

Replace any product containing ingredients considered unsafe with a non-toxic product containing natural ingredients. The fewer ingredients a product contains, the better.

This site has wonderful choices for safe personal care products: http://www.aubrey-organics.com/. For example, the ingredients in Aubrey's Rosa Mosqueta hand lotion are literally good enough to eat!

List all the personal care products – soap, toothpaste, shampoo, body lotion, etc. – you use regularly. Check the ingredient list to see what's in them. You may be surprised to learn that most of the ingredient names are unrecognizable. This is often a bad sign.

Check out a few web sites that list personal care products and their ingredients. Some sites actually rate products by name in terms of their toxicity level. Skin Deep – a project of the Environmental Working Group – has an amazingly detailed and comprehensive site that assists consumers in making healthy, safe product choices: http://www.cosmeticsdatabase.com/splash.php?URI=%2Findex.php

## Toxins to Avoid.

**Phthalates** – a plasticizer used in numerous cosmetics and personal care products and known to damage female and male reproductive organs. Phthalates are associated with hormonal imbalances; damage to the developing testes, as well as the liver, kidneys, and lungs; and allergies.

**Paraben** – a regular cosmetic preservative and common toxin in personal care products, there is serious concern over the long-term impact this toxin has on the human hormonal system. Paraben is an estrogen compound capable of mimicking estrogen activity once it is absorbed into the body.

Other ingredients to steer clear of include, coal tar hair dye – linked to bladder cancer and immune system damage; alpha hydroxy acids – may lead to increased skin cancer risk; and fragrance – which can be comprised of hundreds of individual ingredients, many of which are common human allergens.

## What Else Can You Do?

Strive to make your work and home environments toxic-free. Make little changes to the way you approach your place of work and your household activities:

- If it is necessary to be exposed to industrial byproducts at work or at home, do so in a well-ventilated area and wear a face mask when working with chemicals, including paints and other home repair products.

- Take off your shoes at home. Barefoot is best; leave the lead, pesticides, and dirt on the bottom of your shoes instead of tracking them into your home.
- Carpeting can hold onto toxins – the carpet itself, depending on what it's made from, can be toxic. If possible, lay down rugs made of natural fibers such as cotton and wool, and replace wall-to-wall carpeting with hardwood or ceramic tiles.
- Treat yourself to green plants indoors. They're natural air detoxifiers. Toss out the spray fresheners; remove odors with baking soda, and buy fresh flowers and herbs for fragrance. And invest in a portable air purifier.
- Avoid using pesticides on your lawn and plants.
- Buy food grown using Certified Organic Methods. Avoid food that has been genetically modified or engineered (GMOs). Nearly all processed food contains GMOs.
- Eat a variety of fruits, vegetables, and grains. Specific pesticides are used for specific crops. Eating a variety of food prevents ingesting the pesticide residues a particular food may carry.
- Read food labels. If you don't know what a word means, or cannot pronounce it, don't eat it. Always opt for real food over processed, junk, or fake.
- Review our fertility tips article with specific tips for men women.

# *Pregnancy*

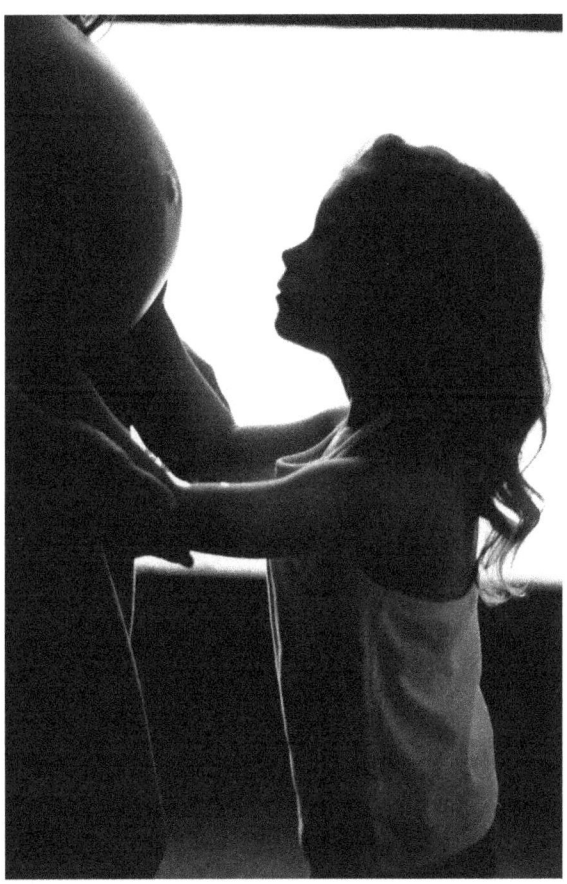

Photography in this chapter provided by Shea Anne at sheaanne.com

According to the Journey to Parenthood via Childbirth Connection.org, *the first trimester is the most important time for mom and her baby. All of the major body systems are formed, and her body and emotions are quickly changing. It is important to evaluate her lifestyle habits and choices to make sure they are in the best interest of her and her baby.*

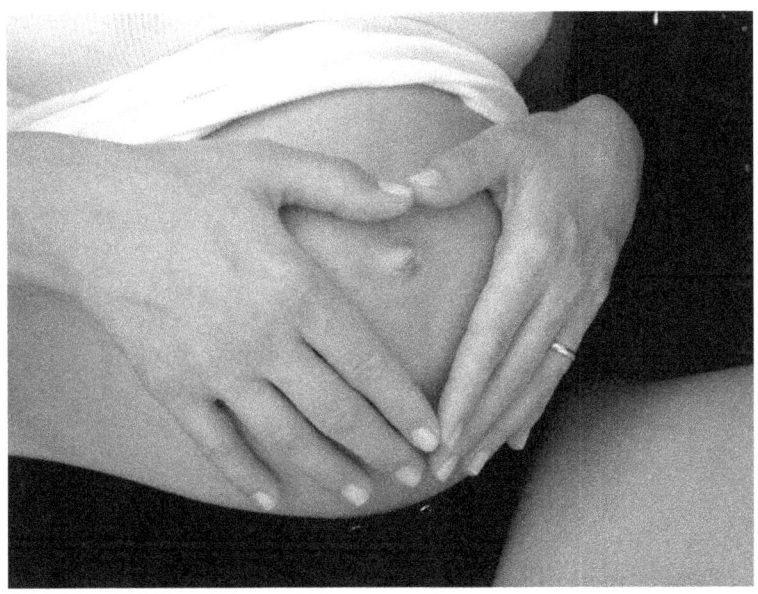

As pregnancy progresses beyond the first trimester, it will remain just as important for a pregnant woman to continue to evaluate her lifestyle habits and diet choices in the best interest of herself and her baby. Pregnancy affects her body and her baby. What she puts in her body and on her skin affects her baby. Her environment affects her body and her baby. According to the Centers for Disease Control and Prevention, *man-made chemicals collect in our bodies, leading pregnant women to worry about what may be reaching their unborn children. Fortunately, you can take simple steps to reduce these risks by being smart about what you eat, drink and breathe.*

Pregnancy is also a sensitive time, a vulnerable time, and one of the most powerful times to:

- Learn or Discover
- Connect

- Heal
- Let Go of Stress or Anxiety
- Ask for Support
- Open up to unlimited possibilities
- Know Your Options
- Prepare
- Go Green

## Learn or Discover

When most of us think about learning or discovering, we often envision taking in as much information as possible through research from books, magazines, online, friends, family, doctors, midwives, maternity consultants and so on. As discussed in chapter two, much discovered or learned during this time, can also bring forth anxiety, fear, and frustration, as pregnancy is treated more like a medical condition by the majority of our culture than it is just a natural human occurrence. There is no question that education and preparation are necessary and important. But there is another kind of learning and discovery that happens during pregnancy and it comes from our body and our baby.

Our body speaks to us. It sends us messages, informing us of many things. By tuning in to our body during pregnancy, we can learn and discover so much about ourselves and our baby. As a result you can strengthen your intuition and as we have discussed earlier in this book, your intuition is a very powerful tool.

Although your baby is in the process of still developing in your womb, your baby also speaks to you. To some this may sound a bit strange, but a mother who tunes in knows, that a baby is just as much alive in her womb as is out of her womb and is absorbing and learning everything mom is going through. As you learn and discover the messages coming from your body and baby during this time, you encourage a deep connection.

## Connect

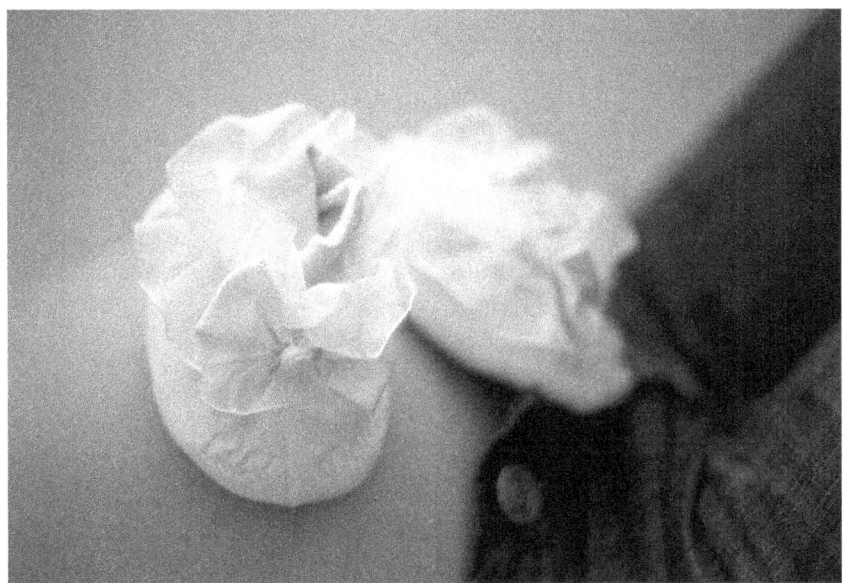

With today's technological advancements, it is pretty easy to connect to everyone and everything around the world, but the most important connection you will have throughout your pregnancy is to your body and your baby, so it is important you take the time to connect. During your pregnancy, invite space so you can take the time to connect with your body and baby. How do you that? Well, begin with taking time to reflect. Put everything aside, even if it's just for five or ten minutes a day to just simply feel your body and feel your baby. No need for instructions or any specific techniques other than just simply remaining present with your feelings. You may be surprised to discover what arises. Practicing this will also be a great preparation for birth. As feelings arise, some may feel pleasant and some may not. When unpleasant feelings arise, we are being provided with an opportunity to heal.

## Heal

Pregnancy is one most powerful opportunities to heal. A woman's physical and emotional changes allow her to be more vulnerable and open. Past experiences and unresolved issues may arise during this time. They are opportunities to work through emotions or feelings that have been hidden or suppressed. By taking the time and space to heal you can let go of what has been a past burden and prepare to welcome your baby in the most nurturing way.

## Let Go of Stress or Anxiety

Giving birth is our natural birthright, however, that does not mean we also don't have the freedom to experience some fears or doubts. Suppressing such feelings of anxiety and stress can not only take a toll on your body, but on your baby as well. It's important to be aware of your fears, anxieties and stressors —to address them, and let go. Doing so will only improve the health of you and your baby, and the outcome of your birth.

How do stress and anxiety affect a pregnant woman and her baby?

When an expectant mom feels anxious and stressed, her nervous system causes physiological changes in her body. Adrenaline and the stress hormone, cortisol, release into her bloodstream, causing her body to react in a fight-or-flight response. As a result, her digestive system slows down, which prevents essential nutrients from being absorbed into her body and passed on to her baby. Her muscles become very tense, making it difficult to think clearly and relax. These physiological changes can lead to premature labor or even complications during labor.

Babies exposed to a variety of stress hormones, toxins and malnutrition inside the womb may develop a host of problems during their fetal growth and after they are born. Their bodies have to undergo certain biological changes in order to cope with a high-stress environment. In October of 2009, The UK Times reported new research that shows exactly how stress can harm a baby's development, and how that stress can lead to long-term problems.

According to research by Vivette Glover, a professor of perinatal psychobiology, maternal anxiety affects the placenta by reducing the activity of the main barrier enzyme that hinders the hormone cortisol from reaching the fetus. The babies of women who were stressed during pregnancy had lower birth weights, lower IQs, slower cognitive development, and more anxiety than those born to the other women in the study.

## How can women cope, and prevent stress and anxiety?

With both my pregnancies, I found a few things essential to my (and my baby's) well-being.

### Acceptance

I had to accept and feel comfortable with my feelings, and not to try to resist them. It is perfectly normal to have some doubts or fears surrounding labor, especially if you are a first-time parent. Once you allow and invite your feelings to be present, you will be able to take the steps you need to take care of yourself and your baby, while reducing — if not eliminating — stress all together.

### Sleep and Relaxation

I made it a priority to rest. It is so important to make sure you are getting as much sleep as your body needs, as well as taking some down time throughout the day. Your body repairs itself during sleep, and also works to restore any imbalances that are occurring. When you compromise sleep, you become more susceptible to stress, as your immune system has to work harder to maintain proper levels of functioning throughout the day. Also consider taking some down time through a yoga or meditation class, a brisk walk or even by lightening your workload.

### Nutrition

I found that nutrition played a very powerful role in both coping with and the prevention of stress while I was pregnant. Caffeine, sugar and processed foods can trigger stress, so it is best to avoid them. Eat whole, fresh organic foods: fruits, vegetables, protein, and healthy fats that are easy to digest, and contain bio-available nutrients that are especially high in B vitamins and minerals. Exposure to sunshine for a few minutes of day will help your body absorb these nutrients. Food contaminants affecting normal fetus development include heavy metals which can be found in some fish and grain products, pesticides which can be found used on non-organic foods, polychlorinated biphenyals (PCBs) found in plastics, and toxins produced by mold. Of course, be sure to consult your midwife, doctor or nutritionist for your specific dietary needs.

## Ask For Support

I sought support. There is no better to time ask for support than when you are pregnant. It is a time when one may realize that it does take a village to support one another and our children. Whether it be from friends, family, birth professionals, or medical professionals, during this time, connecting with those that inspire us, nurture us, guide and support us, allow us to do the same for ourselves and our baby. As a result, it can open us up to unlimited possibilities.

This could be through an expectant mom's group, a childbirth education class, or a qualified professional — such as a birth doula. By working with a birth doula, or attending a birth education class or expectant mom's group, you can prevent or reduce stress levels dramatically. Birth doulas are trained to provide expectant moms emotional and physical support in preparation for labor, and are also present during labor for support. Childbirth education classes are designed to inform expectant mothers of their options for labor and birth, and prepare them for the journey. An expectant mom's group can also be another great resource, as you will be able to relate to and share all the uncertainties and fears you are going through with other women who are going through the same process.

As a result it is important to ask for support and surround yourself with a nurturing environment. If you have tried everything and find yourself helpless and depressed, it's always best to seek help from a qualified professional. There are many professionals who are dedicated and committed to supporting you through your journey, and can provide you and your little one on board with the necessary help.

## Opening Up to Unlimited Possibilities

When we allow ourselves to learn and discover from our own body and baby, connect to our body and baby, heal, and ask for support, it becomes easy to open up to unlimited possibilities. Well, what are those unlimited possibilities you may ask? The possibilities are endless.

Below are just a few:
- A fearless pregnancy
- A joyful pregnancy

- A celebration and appreciation for what your body was naturally designed to do
- Confidence during your labor
- An acceptance of all that comes your way
- A strength and power you were not previously aware was within you

## Know Your Options

During pregnancy it is not uncommon to feel overwhelmed by the advice and experiences given by family, friends, doctors, midwives, childbirth educators etc. There are a lot of decisions to make and everyone seems to have an opinion about what they feel is best for you, from the location of your birth, your birthing method, to your parenting style, but at the end of the day, what is important is what you feel and decide is best for you. With so much information and options available, it is vital to know all your options in order to make informed decisions. Take the time and space to research and decide what will work best for your circumstances, situation, and family dynamics. ChoicesinChildbirth.org provides a National Healthy Guide which you can download from their website. Their website also provides a wealth of information and resources.

If you are limited on time or find yourself overwhelmed and stressed, working with a baby planner may be a great option. Baby Planners are maternity consultants who provide preconceiving, expecting, and new families with unbiased education, resources, and support in all aspects of pregnancy so that you can know all your options and make informed decisions. To find a certified professional baby planner, visit maternityinstitute.com.

## Prepare

Once you know all your options and have made informed decisions about your pregnancy and birth, preparation is essential. This includes creating your own birth plan. A birth plan is an extremely helpful tool for you and others involved in your pregnancy and birth. It clarifies your vision, needs, wants, and also communicates this with your care provider. Two great resources for birth plan samples and birth preparation are prepforbirth.com and birthingnaturally.net.

## Go Green

There is no better time to go green than when you are pregnant. Once you have developed a strong intuition and established a strong connection with your body, it is not that difficult to go green. One of the great gifts of pregnancy is having a physical sensitivity and awareness of the things that make your body feel good and bad. For example your sense of smell is heightened, you may experience cravings, your emotions are heightened, your sense of awareness increases, and so on.

Consulting with a Greenproofer or Greenbirth Educator may be a very useful and rewarding option. They offer guidance, support, preparation, resources, education, and a variety of options.

## What is Greenproofing?

Just as babyproofing is designed to prevent children from injuring themselves or doing damage around the home, a certified greenproofer™ is a maternity eco-consultant that meets with preconceiving, expecting or new families to provide education, support, and resources in order to protect families and their children from unsafe exposure to potentially toxic substances in their home, on their body, and in their environment. Below is an example of a few of the services they can offer:

Home Safety Analysis, Work Safety Analysis, Lifestyle Analysis, Nutrition, Product Awareness, Labor Environment, Nursery Design and Safety, Playroom Safety, Fertility, Pregnancy, Postpartum and Newborn Care, Skin and Body Care, Green Product Selection, Green Child Care Search, Holistic Practitioner Resources , Green Education Classes, Healthy Living Classes, Stress Management, GreenBirth ™ Educator Classes and much more.

To find a certified Greenproofer or Greenbirth Educator near you, visit maternityinstitute.com.

## Tips for Going Green during Pregnancy

- Follow the Green Body Green Birth 4 R's
- Nourish your body and your baby with clean air, food, water, sunshine, sleep, exercise, and stress management
- Know What's in Your Products
- Know How to Read Labels
- Choose Non-Toxic Products
- Avoid Fragrance
- Reduce Electromagnetic fields
- Reduce Stress
- Choose Organic Fresh Food &Clothing
- Prepare Body, Mind, and Spirit
- Prepare a Non-Toxic Home and Work Environment
- Leave Shoes at the Door
- Have a Green Baby Shower
- Create a Green Registry
- Green Your Labor Environment
- Reduce/Eliminate Use of Plastics
- Consume Less (Follow the 4R's of Waste Management)

## Additional Tips:

- Your informed choices can make a big difference for your health, your baby, the health of everyone, and the environment.
- Green does not mean extreme. Small changes add up! Any change can protect you, your baby, and the world your baby will grow up in.
- You have the power to make a difference! Green encourages efficiency, simplicity, and saves you money.

- It is time to celebrate, embrace your body, your baby, and the environment around you.

# Birth & Postpartum

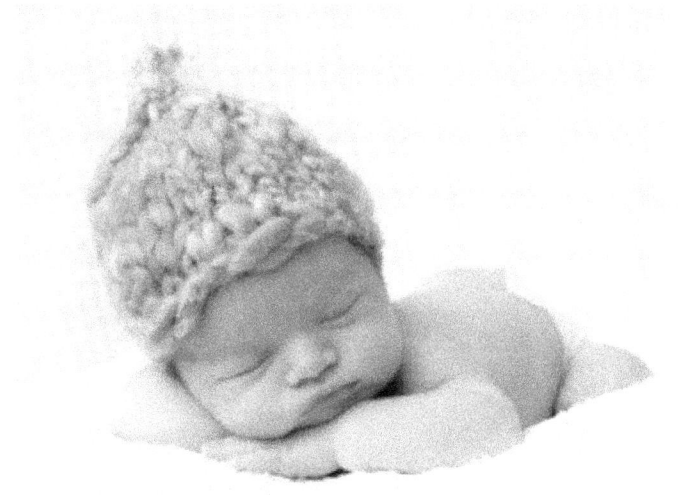

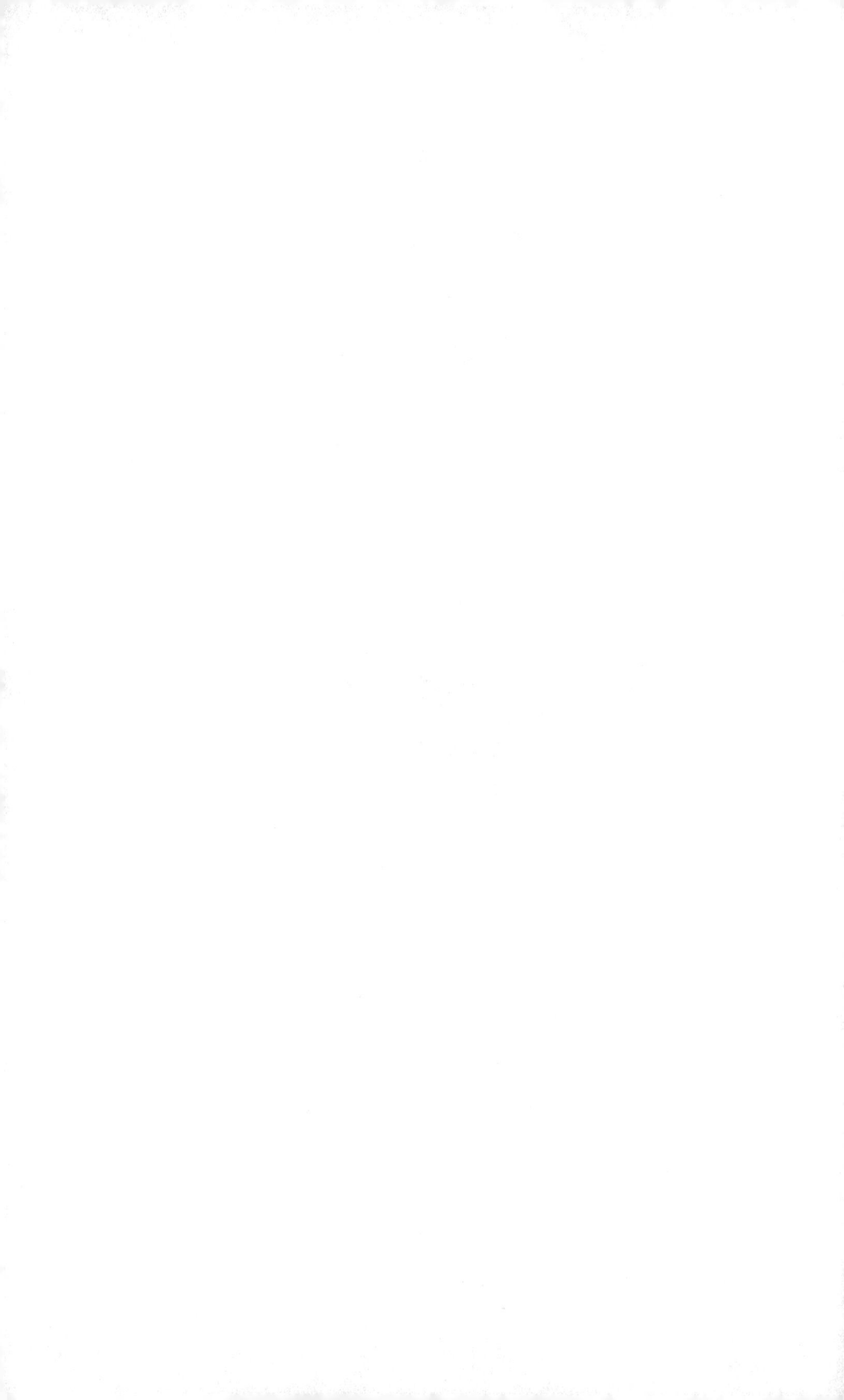

# Preparing for Birth: A Green Labor

As mentioned in the previous chapter, knowing all your options so you can make an informed decision, especially when it comes to where and how you are going to deliver your baby is essential.

Whether deciding to have your baby at the hospital, birthing center, or at home, it is important to consider your labor environment.

Greening a Labor Environment-What to consider:
- Indoor air quality
- Water Quality
- Food Quality
- Clothing Quality
- Lighting
- Sound
- Flooring
- Bedding materials
- Window Treatments
- Non-Toxic Cleaning Products
- Non-Toxic Skin Care Products
- Fragrance Free
- Feeling supported and safe: reusing and recycling your own emotions of intuition and power.

## Hospital

Can a hospital provide a green environment?

It absolutely can and in fact The Deirdre Imus Environmental Health Center ™ at Hackensack University Medical Center (HUMC) represents one of the first hospital-based programs whose specific mission is to identify, control and ultimately prevent toxic exposures in the environment that threaten our children's health. Hackensack University Medical Center was also one of the first in the country to adopt "green cleaning" practices.

Boston's Brigham and Women's Hospital's Shapiro Cardiovascular Center uses only nontoxic cleaners, has banned latex gloves to prevent allergies among workers, and 75 percent of the building's interior is exposed to natural light. Natural light not only reduces energy costs, but scientific studies conducted in the health care sector support the conclusion that natural daylight shortens patient recovery times, improves their mood, and generally promotes well-being.

## Birthing Center

Birthing Centers have also welcomed a green environment. The Taos Birthing Center in New Mexico is one such example.

The Taos Birthship project allows the Birth Center to grow green, offer more to the community and teach more people about natural childbirth, in a completely 'green' building. A sustainable home is an ideal environment for natural childbirth, supporting the family with a Natural and Comfortable Environment in which to give birth.

Another example is the New Birth Company in Kansas. They believe in using their resources well and being good stewards of their bodies, environment and families. Using natural products and avoiding toxins promotes healthy living, healthy community and healthy environment. Simply stated, they believe in natural birth. Less intervention, less materials, less contrived substances, more natural, local products with ingredients they recognize.

## Homebirth

Homebirths provide families the ultimate and most natural opportunity to take control and responsibility over their labor environment. What is important is planning and preparing ahead of time. To ensure a green labor environment, it is important to address and evaluate the components in greening your labor environment as listed on the previous page especially when choosing the place of labor in your home. In addition it is important to have a backup plan and know all your options should you need to be transferred to a hospital for any reason. Visit your backup hospital, and in addition to learning if they are supportive or not of your birth plan and vision, find out how environmentally friendly they are as well. You may find that you may be limited in some of your options and choices, however at least you'll be prepared ahead of time and you can work with your midwife and/or birth doula to come up with some alternative and creative solutions.

## Birth: Welcoming a New life

Just as birth welcomes a new life, it also represents a new beginning for parents as well. Whether you are a first time parent or veteran parent, welcoming a new life will involve the following:

- Inviting the New
- Adapting to Change/Transitions/Adjustments
- Exploration and Learning
- Awareness
- Maintaining Connection
- Letting Go
- A time for unity, support, and collaboration
- Development (not just for infants but ourselves)
- Having a Plan

## Postpartum

Postpartum is a crucial time to invite recovery and support. Mothers often place a lot of pressure on themselves to return back to their normal day to day tasks as well having high expectations about returning to their previous weight, social activities, and so on. During this time it is important to be well equipped and prepared in order nourish yourself and your baby with the best. Prior to birth you may want to put together a plan that includes the following:

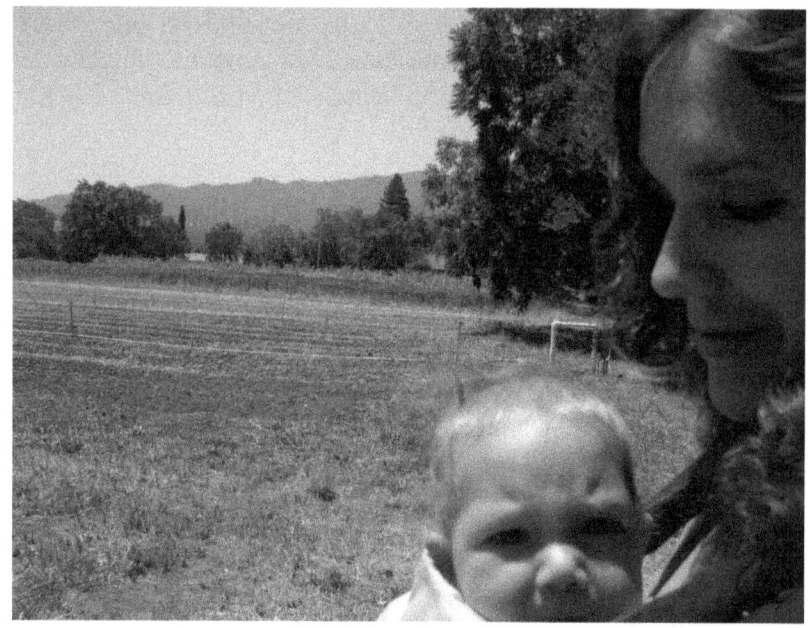

- A recovery plan
- Your postpartum vision/expectations
- Your personal goals
- Your family's goals
- Partner's expectations and roles
- Your support system
- Sleep management
- Stress management
- Child Care management
- Household management
- Work management
- Self-care and time management

Valerie Lynn- McDonough, author of **The Mommy Plan,** and founder of Postpartum Wellness, specializes in traditional post-pregnancy recuperation methods. Below I have included her article, *What?! You don't have a "Mommy Plan" for postnatal recovery? ;*

*As* it emphasizes the importance of a woman's physical and emotional well-being during postpartum.

## What?! You don't have a "Mommy Plan" for postnatal recovery?

By Valerie Lynn-McDonough

Pregnancy and birth have always been a magical time for. Mothers, be it for the first time or for successive children.

Most Mommies planning for a new baby have a Birth Plan, all Moms have a Baby Plan, but a majority of Moms don't have *a Mommy Plan, a plan that focuses on YOU,* a plan for the days and weeks that follows child birth that keeps you on the track for a balanced recovery physically, hormonally and spiritually.

I'm not sure most women realize the chaos our bodies are thrown in while it goes through the natural healing process of reverting back to its pre-natal state in the days and weeks following delivery. Early intervention can make all the difference in having a balanced recovery from child birth or possibly emotional mood disorders that are affect 80% of all women after giving birth.

### First, let's review what is in a typical Birth Plan

A Birth Plan normally consists of the Mommy's preferences. Choice of: doctor, hospital or home birth, mid-wife or doula care, antenatal classes, monitoring of the baby's heart rate via electronic monitoring with belt strapped around you or intermittently via hand held device, atmosphere of the birthing room: e.g. lighting, music, TV, the usage of pain management medication: pethidine, epidural or nothing, birthing companion, positions for labor and birth, assisted delivery or not: forceps or ventous, delivery of the placenta, whether or not the cord blood is stored, feeding the baby: breast or bottle AND any unexpected situations if the baby needs special care.

### The Baby Plan

The Baby Plan contains all the preparation we undertake, including the purchases and changes we get ready our home, and our lives, to welcome our new little bundle of joy. For a first time Mommy a department or specialty store will have an extensive baby registration form all ready for us to fill out so we don't forget any baby necessities and even those baby items we never even knew existed, such as a "wipey warmer!" That was something I never knew existed but did come in handy.

### The Mommy Plan

This plan focuses on two (2) aspects.
- Pregnancy
- Postpartum Recovery

Both periods are very important, however MOST women FAIL TO PLAN for a "balanced" hormonal and physical recover from childbirth.

## PREGNANCY

A woman's body is created to provide the perfect environment for the development of a healthy baby. However, many aspects of our modern lifestyle may affect the baby's development. These include stress, worry, poor dietary habits, sedentary lifestyle and a polluted environment. As mother and baby are a single unit during pregnancy, whatever the mother does to herself will directly affect the baby. One of the most important aspects is adequate nutrition. A pregnant mother must incorporate nutritious food into her diet, for both herself and the baby.

Besides taking care of her health, a pregnant mother should also take care of her emotions. It is a common cultural belief that a pregnant mother who is always unhappy and in low spirit is susceptible to postnatal blues.

### How does your body change?

During pregnancy a Mommy's body goes through a profound transformation where virtually every part is affected:
- Cardiovascular: the amount of blood the heart pumps increases along with your heart rate.

- Breathing: more oxygen is inhaled and extra carbon dioxide is exhaled as a result from breathing for two (2).
- Blood: The amount of blood increases to regulate the body's core temperature to keep the baby's environment at a comfortable temperature.
- Hormones: Estrogen and progesterone hormones increase and;
- Thyroid gland enlarges and the metabolism speeds up.

## How does your anatomy change?

As a baby grows a Mommy's anatomy changes along with it:
- Ligaments and cartilage loosen because of the hormone relaxin.
- Ribs, pelvis and other joints expand to accommodation a growing waist.
- Back pain may occur due to postural distortions.
- Feet, ankles and knee alignment may have also shifted to adapt to postural is changes.

## Persistence of Hormonal imbalance for months

The hormonal changes that occurred during pregnancy persist for months afterward. The period from delivery to the point when the reproduction organs return to a non-pregnant state is known as the postpartum period. A new mother is more fragile than she thinks and has special needs during this short, but critical, time period from the day she gives birth up to approximately 100 days will exist that need to be understood and factored into the recovering weeks of a new-Mom's life.

## Baby Blues vs. Postpartum Depression

The "Baby Blues" are a passing state of heightened emotions that occurs in about half of women who have recently given birth.

After childbirth it is normal to have heightened emotions, such as feeling overwhelmed, on edge, sad, and irritable as hormones are significantly re-balancing during this period. A woman with the Baby

Blues may cry more easily than usual and may have trouble sleeping. This state peaks 3 - 5 days after delivery and lasts from several days to 2 weeks. The Blues DOES NOT interfere with a woman's ability to care for her baby and are so common and expected, they are not considered an illness. However if such feelings persist, it is NOT normal and you should confide in someone and seriously consider to contact your doctor.

For most women, the symptoms are mild and go away on their own. But 10 - 20% of women develop a more disabling form of mood disorder called Postpartum Depression.

### Postpartum Depression Causes

No specific cause of postpartum depression has been found, however hormone imbalance is thought to play a role. Levels of the hormones estrogen, progesterone, and cortisol fall dramatically within 48 hours after delivery. Women who go on to develop postpartum depression may be more sensitive to these hormonal changes.

Don't brush off these feelings - do your own research on the internet. You shouldn't be embarrassed or ashamed if you feel unstable and it is better to get help, which will ultimately help your newborn child and your family. The tendency to develop postpartum blues is unrelated to a previous mental illness and is not caused by stress. However, stress and a history of depression may influence whether the blues go on to become major depression. If you ignore persistent negative emotions they may get worse and could lead to Postpartum Depression, which is way too common in the U.S.

## POSTPARTUM RECOVERY

Having a recovery plan in place may reduce the probability of being affected by pregnancy related mood disorders which strikes 1 in 8 women, or 80%. Pregnant Mommies need to make a plan for themselves for the postpartum recovery period BEFORE they give birth.

After birth, with time, a woman's body (mostly) reverts back to normal; however it's important to optimize the recovery process by understanding the weakened state of your postpartum body. Ten (10) months of pregnancy is taxing on a woman's body and we take care of our body by taking supplements and making adjustments in our diet because we are in essence taking care of our unborn child. Now that we've given birth women must understand that we aren't finished taking care of our body because at this point our body is going through an intense healing process. At this stage our body is still in an "imbalanced" state (Humoral Theory - Hot vs. Cold state) from blood loss and as the body releases excess water, air, fat, toxins and hormones to return itself, physically and mentally, to its pre-baby state.

This is why a Mommy Plan for the postpartum healing period is a must to ensure a "balanced recovery" from childbirth takes place. This is precious time, and we must help our body to heal. No one but you is going to know how you are feeling emotionally and physically. A woman must pay close attention to her feelings during this period. If you are feeling down for an extended time a red flag should go up.

## American culture needs a paradigm shift

American culture emphasizes the preparation period up until the baby is born and then the focus is on the baby, the Mother is secondary. American culture needs to have a paradigm shift and realize that it is vital for a new Mom to take care of her healing body as it reverts to its pre-baby state which again wreaks havoc on our hormones. A woman is pregnant for 10 months, but the human body has the capability to heal itself in approximately 6 weeks or 42 days. However most women don't allow themselves the time needed to recover and push themselves to function "normally" as during their pre-baby life.

In many Asian, Latin American, African and Middle Eastern cultures emphasis is placed on both the new baby and the recovery of the Mother. There are specific traditional, herbal remedies and recipes that have been used for thousands of years to help a new Mother in healing and recovering in a "hormonally balanced" manner in a relatively short time period, 44 days or roughly 6 weeks. Such postnatal recovery products are widely used and readily available with only the application process modernized through technology and ready to use single applications but the formula unchanged.

### The womb is a woman's life force

An Asian belief is that the womb is a women's life force and affects her overall health. Thus the recovery of a woman's womb is very important as it factors into both physical health and energy levels are regained. It is also believed that if a woman doesn't take care of her body after child birth that she will have years of bad health.

### Therefore in your Mommy Plan: Postpartum Recovery:

- Schedule time out for yourself every day for 44 Days
- Purchase specific postpartum recovery products that help you heal from the "inside out."
- Understand the foods you should avoid and foods you should eat that assist the body it its healing. (Postpartum Precautions)

Explain to the people in your life that you need this time for yourself which will allow you to function effectively in the long run as you take care of your new baby.

### Are American women having an "unbalanced hormonal" recovery?

It is believed that not recovering from childbirth in a "balanced and wholesome" manner may result in negative emotional states labeled by the medical industry as the "Baby Blues" that can result in more serious emotional illnesses such as Postpartum depression which is a chemical imbalance in the brain. The U.S. has one of the highest rates of Postpartum depression in the world, 15%, which out of 4.6 million births in 2009 is approximately 690,000 affected women; the unofficial figure is around 800,000. (US Postnatal Industry Information)

No one plans to have the Baby Blues or worse and no one thinks it can happen to them; however 1 in 8 women suffer from some sort of emotional side effect from child birth. Postnatal recovery products are a preventative measure to lower the risk of having such effects. Don't let this happen to you, be proactive, as only you are responsible for the state of your body and health.

diet because we are in essence taking care of our unborn child. Now to 8 week period from the day you deliver. Schedule time for yourself to relax and administer postnatal recovery products. In the end if you take care and heal yourself in a balanced manner you will be reducing the risk from negative emotional side effects from occurring which will ensure you are there for your new baby not only physically, but also emotionally and spiritually.

You can take some control over what is happening to your body. Planning and precaution is the key.

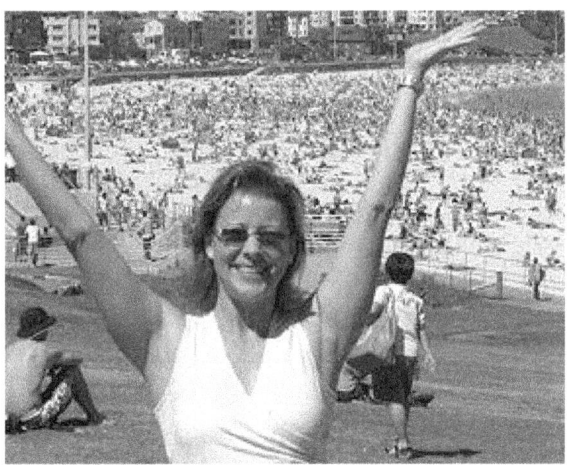

## About Valerie Lynn

Valerie Lynn has been living and working in Malaysia for twelve years. She is the very first foreigner to earn a certificate in Traditional Malay Postnatal Massage in Malaysia. Her passion is traditional post-pregnancy recuperation methods, especially the Malay beliefs and practices.

In addition to being the International Country Coordinator for Malaysia, for Postpartum Support International (PSI) she is a on the Advisory Board for a documentary in the making in the United States called, the After Birth Project. Valerie is also the Chair of the Malay Traditional Postnatal Products and Services Committee for the Malaysian Chamber of Exporters in Kuala Lumpur.

If you are interested in adding the services of a Traditional Post-pregnancy Practitioner to your business or would like to find out more information on the herbal post-pregnancy recovery products, contact Valerie at valerie@postpregnancywellness.com or visit www.postpregnancywellness.com.

## Going Green: Postpartum

It's never too late to begin living a healthier and green lifestyle and postpartum is just as a good a time as any.

A common question often asked is if it is safe to feed baby breast milk because of all the toxins found in mother's breast milk today. I personally feel that the benefit a baby receives from their mother's breast milk outweighs the toxins found in a mother's breast milk.

According to Making Our Milk Safe (MOMS) at safemilk.org:

**If breast milk contains toxins, should I still breast feed?**

ABSOLUTELY! The founders of MOMS each continued to breastfeed their children into the toddler years because they strongly believe in the benefits of breastfeeding to both mother and child. Studies have shown that babies exposed to high levels of PCBs in utero who were subsequently breastfed were less likely than formula-fed babies with similar PCB exposures to exhibit developmental harm as a result of that exposure. In other words, simply being breastfed helped to mitigate toxic exposure that happened in the womb. For this and many other reasons, we believe that continuing to breast feed is the right choice. But toxic chemicals do not belong in our bodies or in our babies. That's why we all need to RAISE OUR VOICES and demand safer chemicals and policies that hold companies accountable for ensuring the products they sell are safe.

Just as we covered in the Pregnancy chapter, very similar tips apply when going green during postpartum:

**Tips for Going Green during Postpartum:**

- Follow the Green Body Green Birth 4 R's
- Nourish your body and your baby with clean air, food, water, sunshine, sleep, exercise, and stress management
- Know What's in Your and Your Baby's Products

- Green Your Baby's Nursery or if Co-Sleeping, Your Bedroom
- Choose Non-Toxic Toys
- Breastfeed
- Know How to Read Labels
- Choose Non-Toxic Products
- Avoid Fragrance
- Reduce EMF's
- Reduce Stress
- Choose Organic & Fresh Food &Clothing
- Prepare Body, Mind, and Spirit
- Prepare a Non-Toxic Home and Work Environment
- Leave Shoes at the Door
- Reduce/Eliminate Use of Plastics
- Consume Less (Follow the 4R's of Waste Management)

**And Remember:**

- Your informed choices can make a big difference for your health, your baby, the health of everyone, and the environment.
- Green does not mean extreme. Small changes add up! Any change can protect you, your baby, and the world your baby will grow up in.
- You have the power to make a difference! Green encourages efficiency, simplicity, and saves you money.
- It is time to celebrate, embrace your body, your baby, and the environment around you.

# *Conclusion*

There is a quote by Julia Cameron, American writer and artist: *"What we focus on, we empower and enlarge"* Rather than placing all of our focus and attention on what to avoid, let's stay focused on the things that nourish us, sustain us, and contribute to our health, well-being and encourage others, through our example, to do the same. By taking care of ourselves, we have more to offer one another and our world.

It's wonderful to see the local and global green movements that are springing up everywhere. It's also wonderful to witness the awareness that is growing with regards to consumerism and the toxic byproducts of that way of life. At the same time there is a vast knowledge of health and well-being growing, and a deep interest of understanding our body and the toxins within. In the birth and parenting communities more and more people and organizations are committed to empowering one another and families to know all their options so they may make informed decisions.

My hope is that this book will give you the desire to harmonize it all, question everything, and point you to that place of hope, empowerment, and peace where one can see that all these movements are beautiful puzzle pieces of one seamless picture where we have the power to contribute to the sustainability of ourselves, one another and our planet.

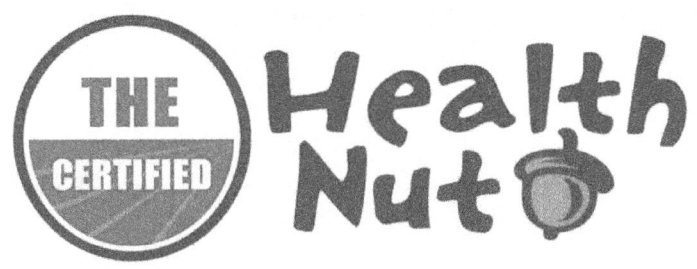

*Green Body Green Birth Spotlight:*

*Troy Casey*

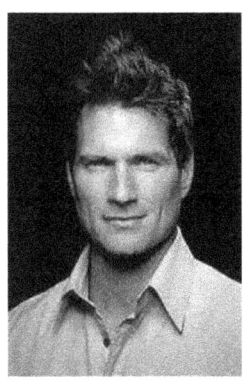
Troy Casey's message is simple: Healthy Me = a Healthy Planet.
This simple message is the very reason I resonate with Troy and his work so deeply.

His mission is teaching holistic health, self-care and our symbiotic relationship to planet Earth in addition to inspiring conscious choices and "voting with YOUR dollars" in order to create a healthy happy world and the future of Mankind.

A few quotes from Troy that I also resonate with and compliments Green Body Green Birth's message:

*"If we are not healthy ourselves, how do we expect the world outside of us to be healthy?"*

*Regarding the expense of buying organic: "Pay Now or Pay Later.... Pay the Farmer or Pay the Doctor!"*

*"Remember: YOU are also the miracle that was a baby!"*

Whether, you resonate with Troy's lifestyle and beliefs or not, one thing you can't help but admire is that he walks the walk. Troy is true living example of what he teaches.

Here is an interview excerpt Troy did with CarbonConscious.us

**Q**. What do you think should be the number one priority for creating healthier lives and a healthier environment?
**A**. Raising consciousness about food and human health. Doing interviews on the street, I realized people understand that what is good for them is good for the earth and vice versa; yet the choices we are presented with on a daily basis do not reflect this.

Most people do not know what GMOs (genetically modified organisms) are or that GMOs are in their food. They are unaware that farming practices of five multinational conglomerates destroy the flora and fauna necessary to continue life on earth. Einstein said, *"If the bee disappeared off the surface of the globe, then man would only have four years of life left. No more bees, no more pollination, no more plants, no more animals, no more man."*

**Q.** It seems that our food and ecosystem have been negatively impacted by the way that we live our lives. Is it sustainable to keep doing what we are doing?
**A.** Absolutely not! Five percent of the world's population using 30 percent of the natural resources contributing to 25 percent of the pollution...statistically that is a failed system, one that cannot be exported to China, India or any developing country. If U.S. leaders do not recognize this and immediately work to subsidize new energy like they subsidize genetically modified organisms in milk, it looks very ugly for us and the planet! At this moment, it appears that politicians do not have a vested interest in this because it is not "economically feasible." I like to quote the Native American Cree proverb: Only when the last tree is cut, the last river is polluted and the last fish is caught will we realize that we can't eat money.

**Q.** Food and climate change are integrally related. Many people see reducing the consumption of meat as the number one way to reduce greenhouse gas emissions. Do you have any thoughts on this?
**A.** I think that factory farming, with its use of hormones and antibiotics and feeding animals GMOs, is harmful to the environment and humans. There is no doubt about the need for respect and reverence for the earth and earthlings, as well as many systems in need of a complete overhaul, yet I feel that many environmentalist agendas are misguided and/or politically driven.

**Q.** Where does one start on bettering the earth or living a more eco-friendly life?
**A.** People need to start with themselves and be healthy! The human being is the first sustainable environment. What is good for humans is good for the earth.

If we are truly concerned about our carbon footprint, why are we not subsidizing solar and wind power or electric cars like we subsidize GMO agribusiness and milk or war and weapons? I see many groups vilifying human beings for their carbon footprint without holistic and sustainable solutions for all. People eat meat and need food; getting them to change something that is part of their DNA is much harder than implementing laws that promote peace.

**Q.** Most people understand that the Amazon rainforest provides the planet with many important environmental benefits. Since you've spent many years studying health and the natural environment, can you speak to the specific environmental attributes of the rainforest that naturally help mitigate climate change?
**A.** About 20 percent of Earth's oxygen, one-third of fresh water and half of all species on the earth come from the Amazon. Because of the oxygen and rain the Amazon produces, it has been called the lungs of the planet and is considered the global cooling center.

Biodiversity is a critical component of our species' survival, and the Amazon is the most bio diverse place on earth. The cure for AIDS, cancer and diabetes is believed to be in the rainforest. I believe that all degenerative diseases can be reversed with the life-giving plants of the rainforest. I am living proof of the efficacious power and longevity potential of these plants; they have improved my strength and clarity of mind immensely. I feel I am regenerating at a cellular level.

**Q.** What is it about the rainforest that offers the elixir to better health?
**A.** Its nutrient-dense herbs and their complex alkaloid structure are unparalleled and unprecedented in any other plants on earth. The Amazon is home to the most powerful life force energy on the planet, the highest concentrated source of vitamin C, the highest concentrated source of antioxidants and of beta carotene, the last virgin soil, the strongest genetic codes, etc. etc. Of the 215,000 Amazonian plant species, only 1 percent of the plants have been studied. The National Cancer Institute has documented 3,000 plants—25 percent of all cancer drugs on the market and 42 percent of all drugs get their impetus from the Amazon.

As we know, drugs have side effects. We have seen the commercials: "erectile dysfunction or even death… ask your doctor if this is right for you." The whole food substances or food-grade medicinal herbs that we use in the Amazon Herb Company product line can be consumed just like foods and they have powerful nutritional value. Hypocrites said, "Let thy food be thy medicine." I believe the creator/god designed the human body to heal itself... if it has the proper nutrition.

**Q.** What can people do to help preserve the rainforest?
**A.** Use sustainable plants, herbs, super foods, nuts and berries harvested by the indigenous tribes. They simply grow back and it empowers the inhabitants to keep the rainforest intact. Eco-tourism is another good idea as it is a sustainable industry that helps create respect and reverence for the jungle. The strongest testament to keeping the rainforest alive and productive is more economically profitable than cutting it down. Our company also funnels 10 percent of the profits back into aceer.org educational programs to teach children the cultural value of their plant knowledge.

**Q.** Do you think we are on our way to better health?
**A.** Yes, although statistics do not reflect that. I have to believe and hold a positive vision of the future because I believe our thoughts create reality. People are slowly shifting to the realization that something is amiss and taking responsibility for their own health is paramount. I hold a clear vision of clean air, water and soil and peace on earth coming very soon.

**Q.** To follow up to that question – what toll has the environment had on Americans' health?
   Current statistics are staggering: we rank 36th in the world for health, 1 in 3 have cancer, 67 percent of Americans are obese, diabetes is at epidemic proportion, autism, Alzheimer's, Parkinson's, chronic fatigue and many other new diseases.
   I believe that the chemical contamination of the air, water and soil have a direct correlation to our health. The previous statistics prove it to me. It is simple common sense—we are in a symbiotic relationship to everything in our environment. I say how do we expect to have a healthy planet unless we ourselves are healthy?

Troy's story is also an inspiration:
   After growing up on the streets as a kid, having drug & alcohol problems as an adult, Troy found solace in the holistic lifestyle and healed himself. Economically motivated as a Versace model in Milan, Italy 22 years ago, Troy started studying internal purification

and nutrition as a holistic way of looking and feeling great in front of the camera. Continuously studying and practicing what he discovered extensively traveling the world, Troy now counsels, lectures and inspires people all over the planet with choices for a healthier life. His specialty is holistic health, Wild Amazonian plant medicine & super foods. Most recently he has worked on Discovery's Planet Green Network and his levity provoking alter ego, Certified Health Nut, can be seen on Youtube.com and CertifiedHealthNut.com

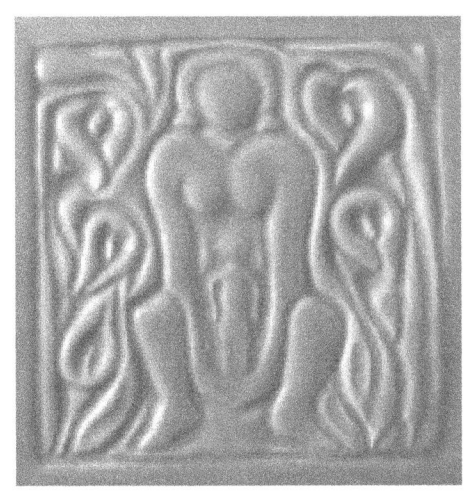

# *ECOBIRTH*

## *By Molly Arthur*

# FORWARD

*by Mary Oscategui*

It is with much pleasure and honor that I introduce to all of you the work of Molly Arthur and the EcoBirth organization. When I first met Molly we connected immediately as we both share a tremendous passion for birth and in particularly its' relationship to the earth.

EcoBirth, Women for Earth and Birth, unites the earth and birth movements for the well-being of our world, wants to ensure that there are no more toxins in our bodies or in our developing babies, and wants our babies born in a caring, natural way and raised in a safe, non-toxic world.

In the next few pages, Molly shares her story through her environmental legacy, mapping and connecting with her environmental lineage.

Mapping and connecting with your environmental lineage not only gives you an opportunity to explore what influences the environment has had on your mother, grandmother, and great-grandmother, but the influences it may also have on your children and grandchildren.

In addition, exploring and connecting with your environmental lineage opens a gateway to have a deeper understanding and compassion for what has happened in your historical ancestry, thus giving you the power to heal, change and influence your current and future lineage.

I have lived in Marin County for over 20 years, raising my family, making a living, growing into myself. It has held me in a beneficence that broods o'r my heart and is manifest in the beautiful Mt Tamalpais. My Grandmother wrote poems at the turn of the century about this decidedly feminine mountain, now I get to still walk on its curving breast and be nurtured. All four of my grandparents lived in San Francisco and raised my parents in The City. My Grandfather used to come to Marin County in the summers at the turn of the century- 1900s- together with his large Irish clan to stay in their wooden, rustic cabin.

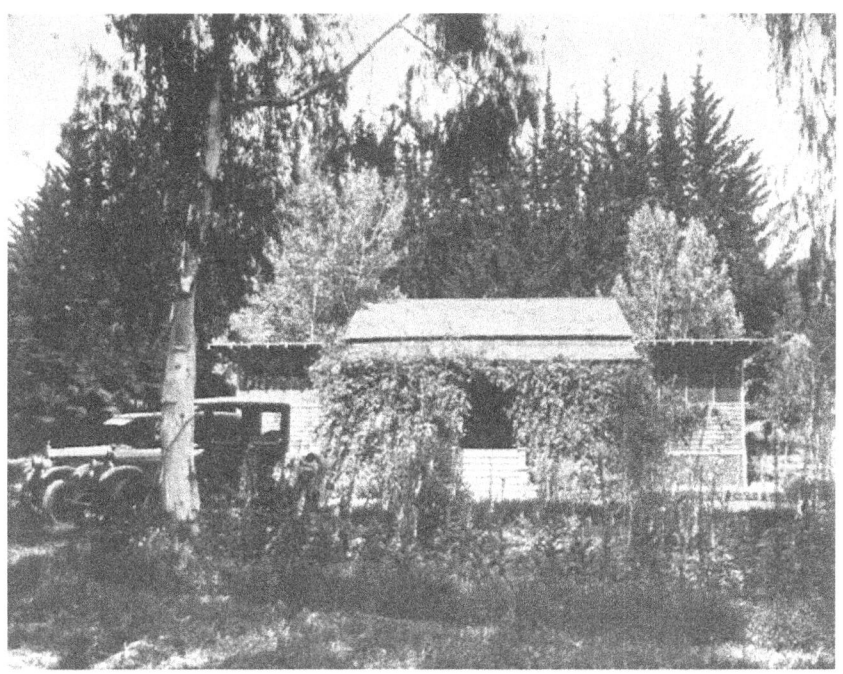

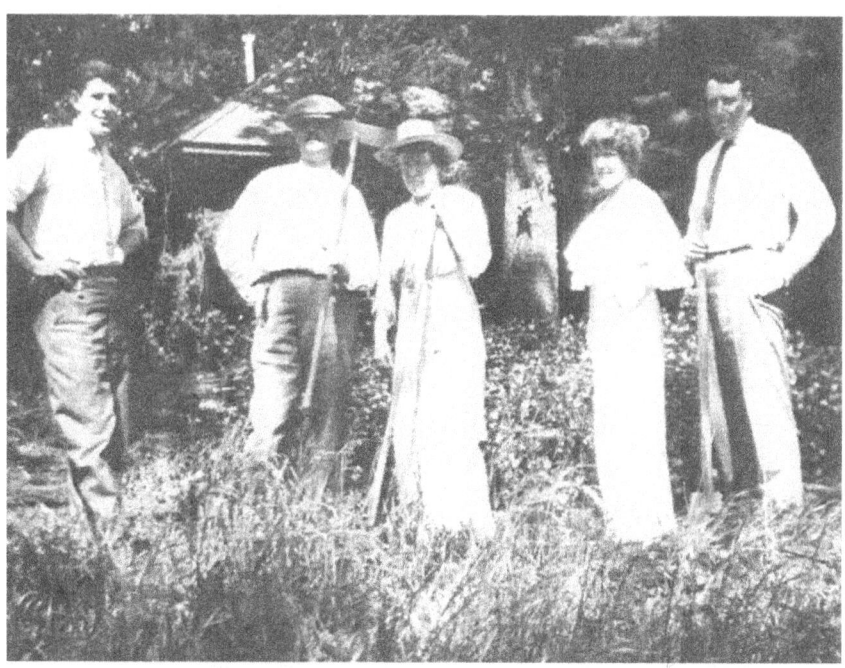

And his side of my family came here after the 1906 San Francisco Earthquake for refuge. He told me of swimming in the local creek in Kentfield.

So I have some strong personal connections to the place where my husband and I raised our two children. And truly it was not so long ago that my relatives felt happy to swim in local creeks, but now I would not let my grandchildren swim in the local creek because of my fear of toxins in it.

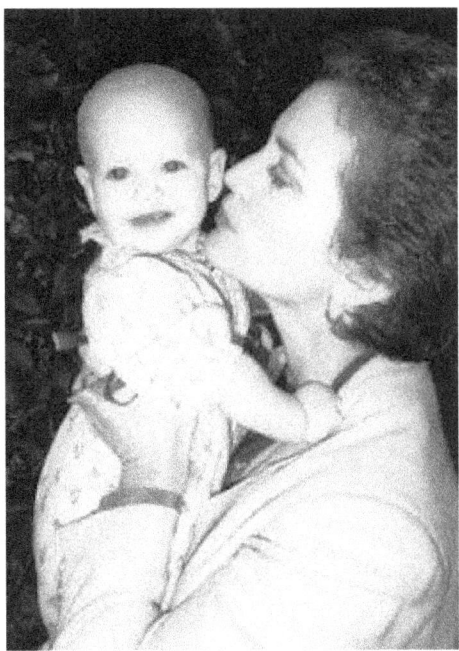

I started thinking about the shape of our world when I was done raising my children and had fulfilled my personally assigned mission of raising them to be good, productive people.

But I noticed that the world had drastically become a worse place for humans and any species to survive and thrive. I became conscious of the ravaging of ourselves and our Mother Earth when I understood that our expectant babies were pre-polluted by our own bodies[1] and that our birthing was dismissed as inherently risky and frightening, rather than nature's way of sacred creation. This is a brief story about my increasing awareness of what is happening to our world, in a very personal way and a growth of my commitment to do something about it.

---

[1] *EWG Report || BodyBurden 2* - The Pollution in Newborns *www.ewg.org/reports/bodyburden2/*study coordinated by the Environmental Working Group that found an average of 200 industrial chemicals and pollutants in umbilical cord blood from 10 babies...

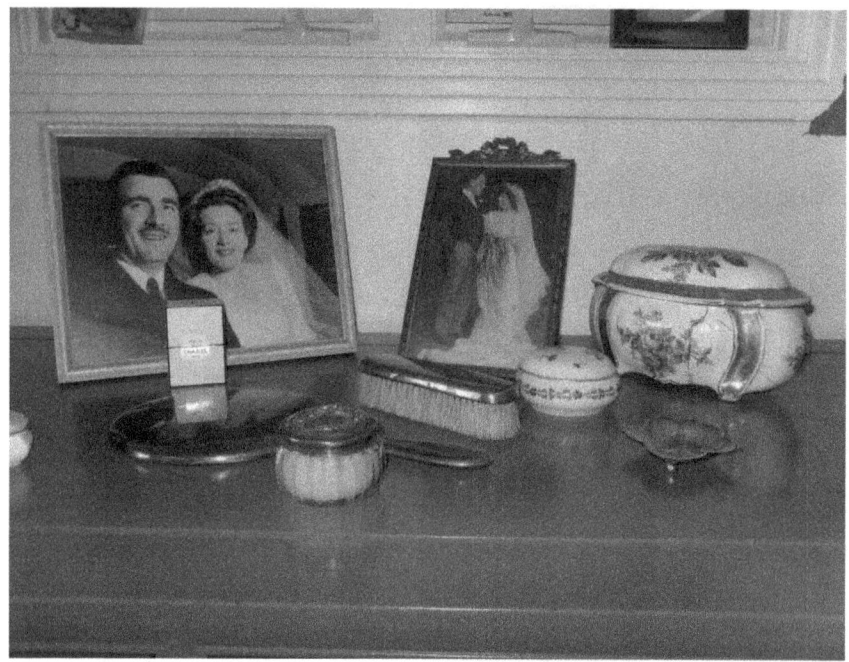

I picked a brochure up at the Fairfax EcoFest a few years ago that said something was wrong with having perfume on our bodies[2]. I thought about the precious perfume bottle that my mother gave me as a "coming of age" acknowledgement which has been on my bureau for decades, really.

But now I understood from this brochure that it contains chemicals that are correlated with cancer and hormone disruption that can affect fetuses, especially in the 1st trimester. When I looked further into it, I found out that Chanel #5[3] was invented in 1921, when my mother was an adolescent and I distinctly remember the lovely smell of it because she used it for her frequent social forays. It is associated with my love for my mother and hers for me, but she had breast cancer when she was 38 and I was just two.

---

[2] http://healthbrochures.info/images/Fragrance%20Facts.pdf
[3] Houlihan J, Brody C, Schwan B. 2002. Not Too Pretty. Environmental Working Group. Available: http://www.ewg.org/reports/nottoopretty

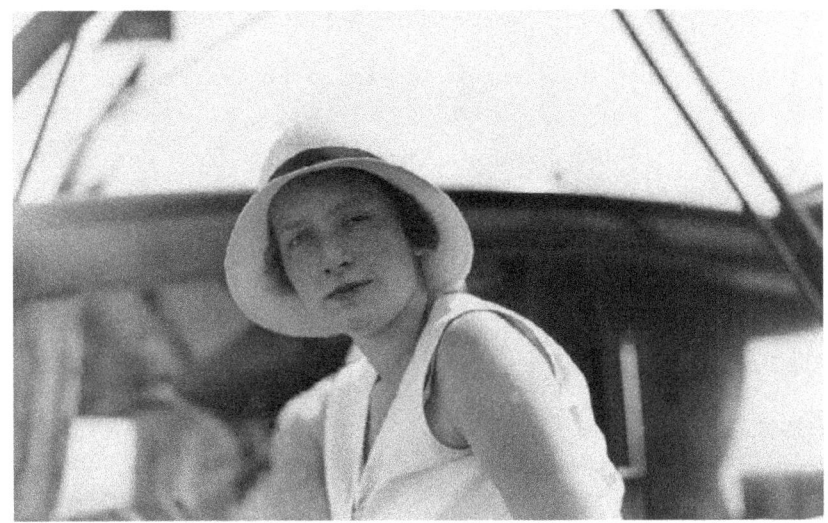

I started wondering about the perfume and my mother's cancer, and then I started wondering about my sister's birth defect of an unformed left hip bone, her early puberty, obesity and death from cancer at age 52. I wanted to learn more about what a hormone disruption[4] was and what it was doing in my mother's body and whether it may have created my sisters bone defect and even had influence on the rest of her vulnerable life story.

My sister, Patty, appeared to be the most beautiful, intelligent, funny and creative member of our extended clan.

---

[4] http://www.endocrinedisruption.com/home.php Colborn T, Dumanoski D, Myers JP. 1996. *Our Stolen Future: Are We Threatening Our Fertility, Intelligence, and Survival?—A Scientific Detective Story.* New York: Dutton.

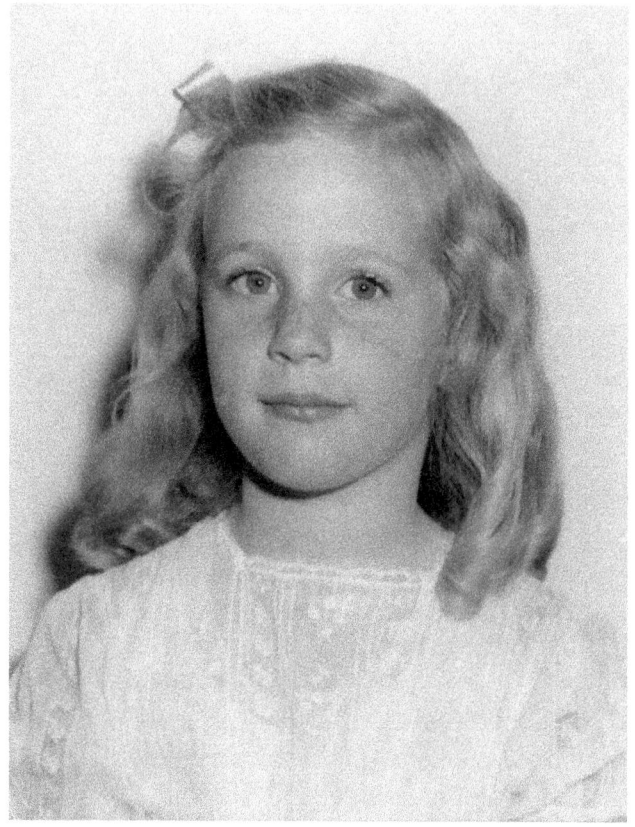

But her potential was stunted and ended much too young. Was it just that my sister had weak self control over her addiction to smoking and food? Or could the involuntary absorption of this particular synthetic chemical (perfume/phthalates)[5] in my mother's life have caused harm to my sister in utero (during WWll, 1945) and

---

[5] Baby boys and pregnant women are two groups especially vulnerable to hormone-disrupting effects of phthalates. Alarmingly, these are precisely the groups whose high level exposure to multiple phthalates has been extensively documented (Adibi 2008; Sathyanarayana 2008; Silva, Barr 2004). Phthalates cross the placenta into amniotic fluid (Silva, Reidy 2004); they are also transferred from the mother to the infant with breast milk (Main 2006). A child's exposure to these potent anti-androgenic chemicals starts from the prenatal stage and continues through the formative early years. As a result, the exposure of children to phthalates generally exceeds that of adults (Heudorf 2007). Infants, with their small body size, and different behavioral patterns from adults, are most at risk from phthalates. http://www.ewg.org/node/26052

impacted her later in life during her puberty and even her adulthood? Then, I realized, obvious! That Patty's and my genesis, our eggs, were actually formed in my grandmother's body, in my mother's body, when my mother was eagerly expected as the first baby of the growing Fay clan[6]. Whew, what was happening in San Francisco in 1912? How do I figure that out?

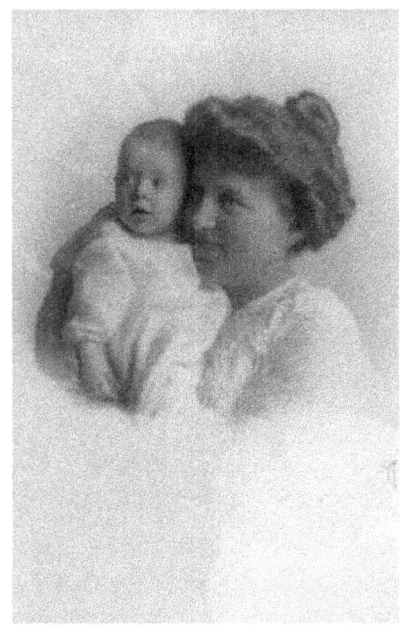

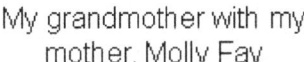
My grandmother with my mother, Molly Fay

I talked to experts involved in environmental health and delved into internet search. I did not have to go far, just to the EPA and other governmental websites- the most documented toxins were heavy

---

[6] Exposure to gene-altering substances, particularly in the womb and shortly after birth, "can lead to increased susceptibility to disease," said Linda S. Birnbaum, Director of the National Institute of Environmental Health Sciences and of the National Toxicology Program. "The susceptibility persists long after the exposure is gone, even decades later. Glands, organs, and systems can be permanently altered. There is a huge potential impact from these exposures, partly because the changes may be inherited across generations. You may be affected by what your mother and grandmother was exposed to during pregnancy," Birnbaum said. Such exposures can disrupt the way that genes behave, according to both animal and human studies. These changes, in turn, can be passed on to the next generations.
http://www.environmentalhealthnews.org/ehs/news/epigenetics-workshop

metals: mercury left over from the Gold Rush mining[7] and lead paint in all our lovely Victorians[8]: very specific results from living right. here in San Francisco. I pulled out our family albums and written histories. Turns out that my male ancestors were involved in Western

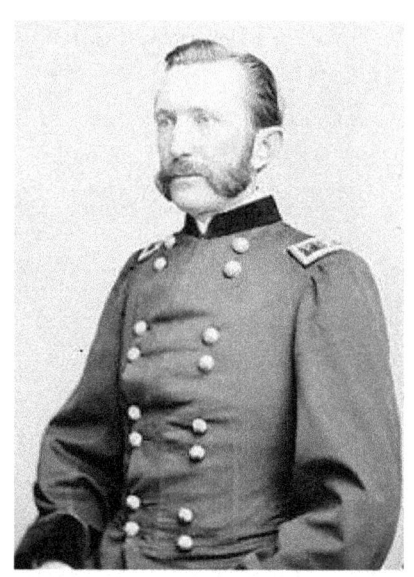

P. Edward Connor

"Father of Mining" in Utah

1863

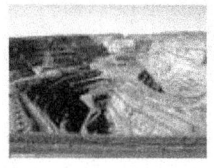

mining[9] and in retail-a paint store in San Francisco in the 1890s! Geez. I was discovering that my heritage was not just genetic but environmental too. Our immutable connection to our ancestors was manifest not only through our genes, like our red hair and freckles,

---

[7] EPA's website on mercury
[8] http://www.leadsafe.org/content/homes_and_lead/
http://www.ewg.org/chemindex/chemicals/22794
http://www.epa.gov/safewater/lead/leadfactsheet.html
[9] http://en.wikipedia.org/wiki/Patrick_Edward_Connor

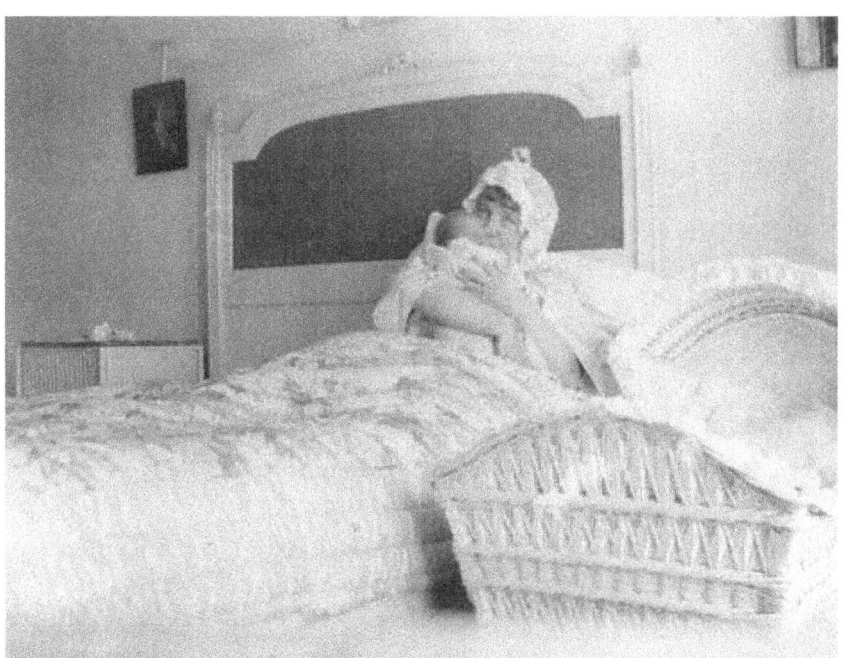

but in our health vulnerabilities and susceptibilities, just because our ancestors were in San Francisco, exposed to the reality of life there and then, which contained mercury and lead toxins.

I still have the crib that my grandmother told me she kept close by the side of her bed so she could pat her babies to sleep, comforting them when they cried. She was given that crib by her mother for her first baby- my mother. My grandmother had 7 babies, but one was a stillbirth, which still grieved her when she and I discussed it when she was in her 80's. Now I realize that that crib was undoubtedly painted with lead paint, -which causes physical and neurological disorders, as

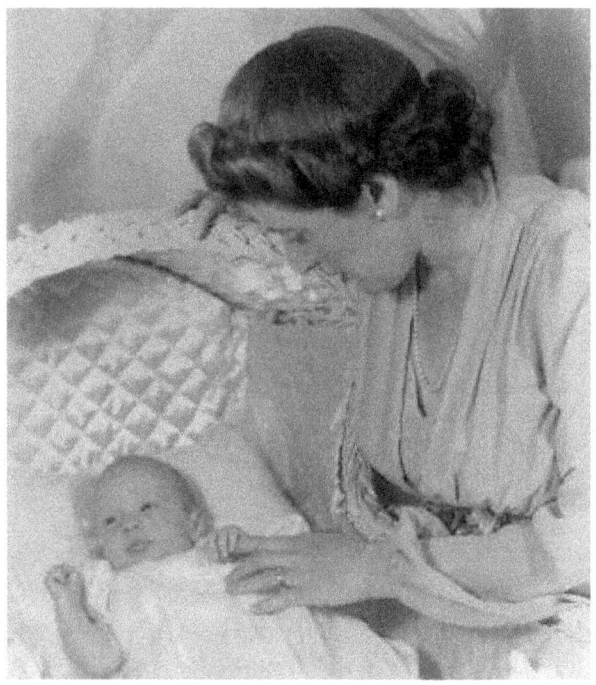

well as behavior, earning and intelligence problems in children. I was rocked in that cradle as an infant too, and it was passed onto me with such love from my mother, who sewed new pink satin lining and bows for my two children embracing sleep in this special, precious heirloom. This crib has come to symbolize to me the adulteration that involuntary poisons can do to our lives, even when we are offering love and connection to our beloved babies.

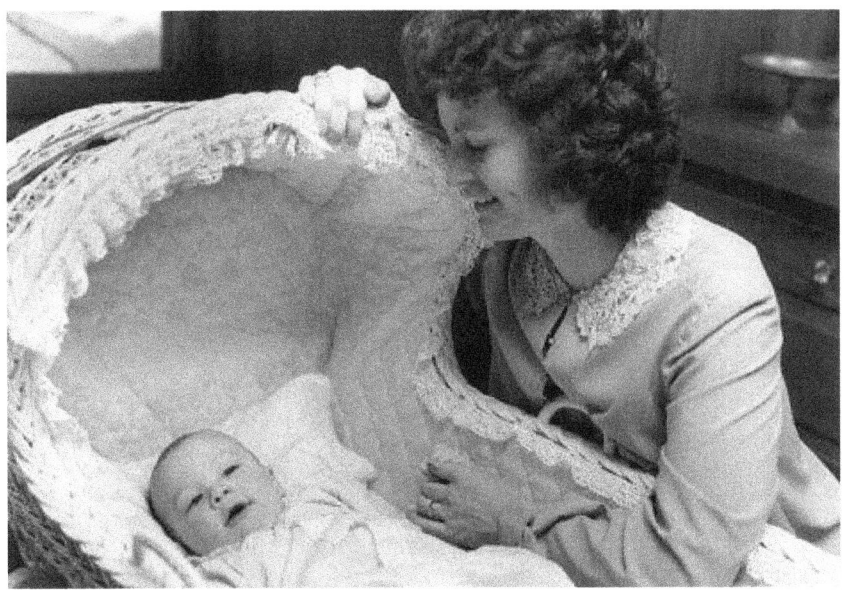

How does this ignorance of harm come to be a part of my lineage- why does my story get corrupted by these inadvertent, unknown substances in my life? I was getting fierce in my search, this was not right, that I was passing onto my children and grandchildren harm that I knew nothing about but had invaded my body and my life.

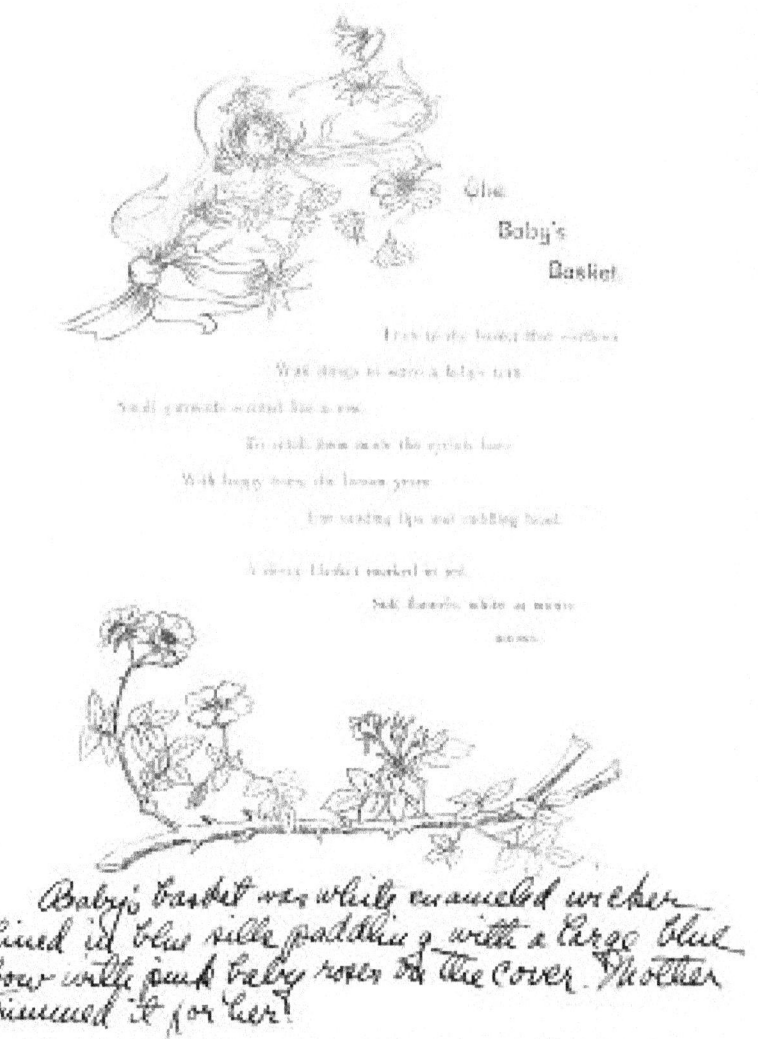

    I wanted to know about how we were birthed too, because I wondered if birthing practices could have just as much effect on our health, as these ubiquitous chemicals, because after all, the first environment is our mother's body, which I thought was pure and unadulterated and now I find is not.

    I read my mother's baby book, a treasure filled with my grandmother's wispy handwriting.

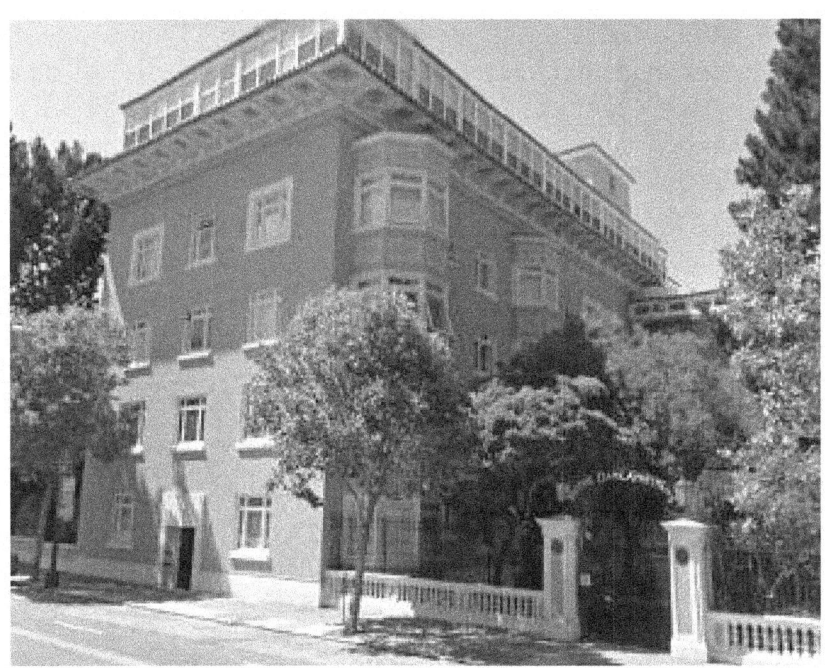

Present day version of Adler Sanitarium

My mother was born in one of the first maternity hospitals in San Francisco, the building is still there (now condos) on Van Ness and Broadway. If chemicals ingested by breathing and drinking could be harmful, what about the drugs given during birth?

Wow, I found out that something called Twilight Sleep[10] was used early in the 1900s, particularly in hospitals, administered by male doctors. So, my guess is that my grandmother received it. I spent some months reading up on the possible implications of drugs and birth practices. I found this study that concluded:

"Adults who met diagnostic criteria for drug addiction were about five times as likely as sibling controls to have received three or more doses of opioid and barbiturate drugs within ten hours before birth."[11]

---

[10] ^ 🌐 "Twilight Sleep". *Collier's New Encyclopedia*. 1921.
[11] (Nyberg, Buka, and Lipsitt 2000). Evidence-Based Maternity Care: "What It Is and What It Can Achieve " Bt Carol Sakala and Maureen P. Corry,Co-published

It appeared that drugs did affect our babies. I know that my mother was "put out" during our births, happily she said, and of course, we were not breastfed, which actually is such a strong basis of connection between mother and baby and an indicator of their future health. So what were we fed, if not the perfectly balanced and evolved nutrition from a mother's body?

---

**MARY'S HELP HOSPITAL**

145 Guerrero St.  San Francisco, Calif.

Phone MArket 0733

Date 3-15-44

For Baby McGettigan

Birth Date 3-5-44  Birth Weight 6 lbs. 10½ oz.

Present Weight 6 lbs. 10 oz. Height 19½ in.

**FEEDING FORMULA**

1. _16_ ounces boiled water (boil 10 minutes)
2. Cool water till warm, then add:
3. _3_ level tablespoons *Dextri-Maltose* (Soluble Carbohydrate)
4. _8_ ounces ~~Irradiated Carnation Milk~~ *Special morning milk*

Pour this formula into _6_ bottles of _4_ ounces each. Cover each bottle with a sterile stopper and keep in a cool place until needed.

Feed baby every _4_ hours, or _6_ times daily.

Hours for feeding 10-2-6 A.M. 10-2-6 P.M.

I found a copy of the take-home instructions given out by the hospital in 1944 on preparing a formula of the right mixture of dextrose maltose and canned, irradiated condensed milk with a note "You may continue to give your baby Irradiated Carnation Milk after weaning from the bottle. The same good qualities which have helped make your baby a strong healthy child will continue to help him through all his growing years".

So ironic, I discovered an old magazine ad displaying lead solder being used in infant formula cans - we were given cow's milk, sugar and lead for our nourishment, instead of the health supporting, immune resistant mother's breast milk. Perhaps my mother's generation of birth practices contributed to the addictions that 80% of my extended family suffers from.

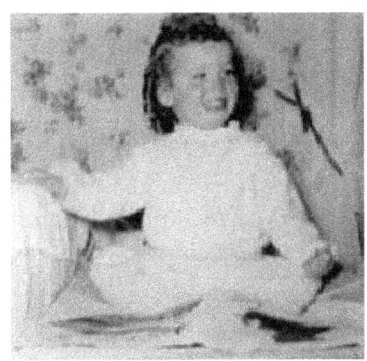
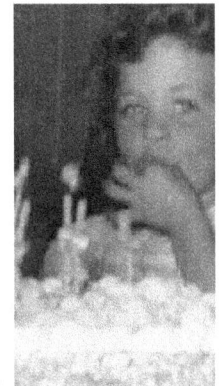
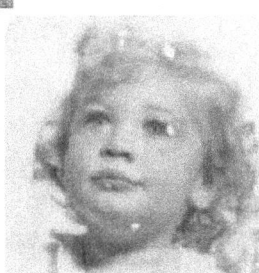

I recently realized that I was addicted to sugar, not surprising really, considering what I ingested from the hazardous cans of baby formula fed to me.

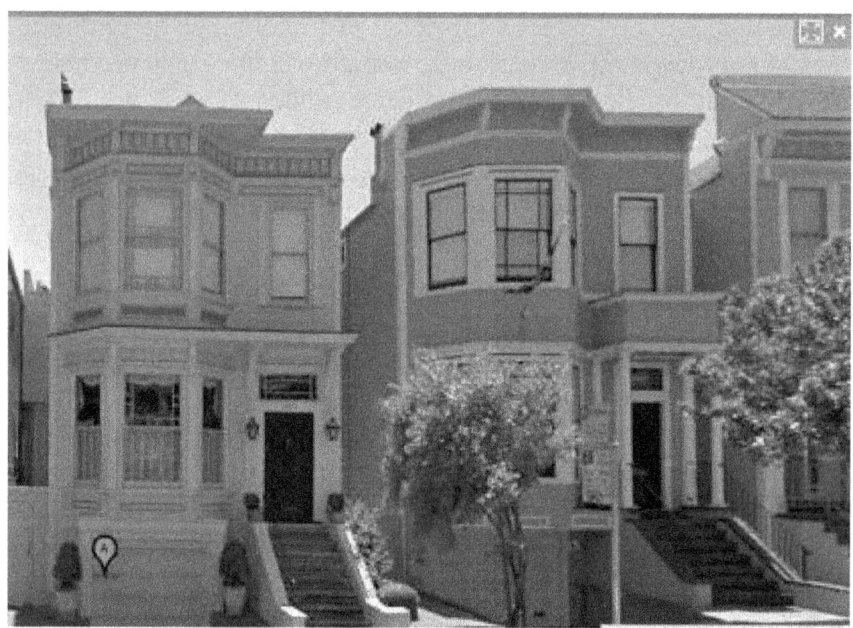

My home was a wonderful San Francisco Victorian, with whistling, shaking windows that let the fog in, and a lot more toxins that increased in the 1950's as a result of the synthetic chemical industry and agri-business development. BPAs,[12] part of the phthalates family of chemicals, were introduced to my home in personal care products such as soap, shampoo, hair spray, deodorants, and fragrances.[2], new household items, marketed through the wonderful little TV box, and in the pesticides that transferred to my body from the vegetables and meat that I ate. We always had cheap meat, bread and frozen vegetables for dinner and a sweet dessert!. The soda I drank could have come from the spring that was used by the local bottling company, just 3 miles from Hunter's Point[13] toxic chemical stew which was dumped until 1970 over the sides of the ships that have been built for war here since WW1. Our old plumbing pipes were probably lead, and the vinyl flooring in our kitchen probably contained phthalates. The accumulation of these toxins in

---

[12] http://healthychild.org/issues/chemical-pop/bisphenol_a/
http://www.sciencenews.org/view/generic/id/48065/title/Science_%2B_the_Public__BPA_in_the_womb_shows_link_to_kids%E2%80%99_behavior

[13] http://cfpub.epa.gov/supercpad/cursites/csitinfo.cfm?id=0902722

my body could have affected whether I could get pregnant and have healthy babies.

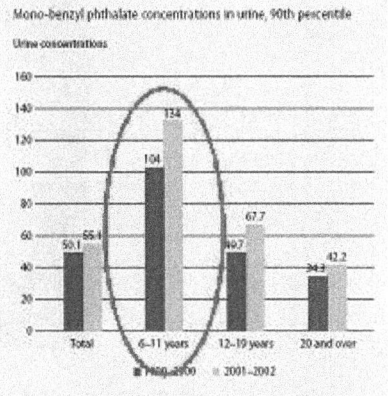

Americans are widely exposed to phthalates

Early life exposure to phthalates holds the greatest risk for harm and prenatal exposure to very low doses can have irreversible, lifelong effects. More recent studies link phthalate exposure to early puberty in girls and suggest that females are affected in other ways that may increase the risk of breast cancer. [14]

---

[14] http://www.breastcancerfund.org/clear-science/chemicals-glossary/phthalates.html

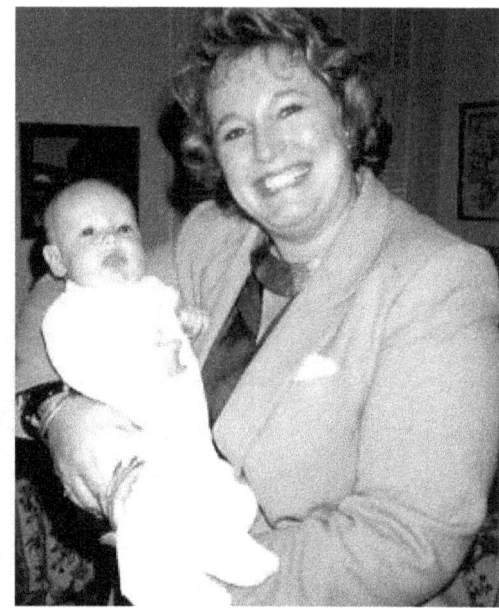

My sister, Aunt Patty and my daughter, 26 years ago.

I was relieved of my anger at my sister at this point, it came to me that it is very possible that her addictions to smoking and food/sugar/flour- her lifestyle choices, were probably not the main reason she had what I considered an unproductive life. It was likely that the influences of her environment in utero, and during our childhood, all involuntary interventions in her natural development, were largely responsible for her vulnerable health, lack of mental resilience and early death by cancer.

I grieved the extinguishing of her bright laughter, ribald humor and wry perspective on life. I miss our belly-laugh times together, remembering our shared family challenges together that were so funny when recounted by her acerbic and outlandish humor.

I learned more about the history of lead in our world and mercury in our ecosystem and the ubiquity of the over 80,000 new synthetic chemicals in our lives.

## Chemical production is rising

U.S. chemical production has increased dramatically over the last 60 years. The number of chemicals registered for commercial use now stands at 80,000—a 30 percent increase since 1979.

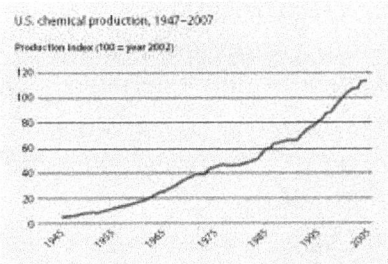

U.S. chemical production, 1947-2007

It appeared to be an old story: that making a living, like my male ancestors did to support their families and pioneer a new land here on furthest Western edge of the US,[15] perpetuated harm to their families, but benefited industries that used complicity and duplicity and plain old criminal acts to prop up their profits. An industry even grew up in the medical care offered to women and babies, which now is associated with over 60% of hospital admissions. [16]What happened to the back to earth birth movement that we promulgated in the 70's and 80? It was eclipsed by an industry that leveraged women's desires to

---

[15] http://fletcherfamilytree.wordpress.com/2009/06/13/denis-j-oliver-diaries/
[16] 1. Sakala C, Corry MP. *Evidence-based Maternity Care: What It Is and What It Can Achieve.* New York: Milbank Memorial Fund, 2008. Available at: www.childbirthconnection.org/ebmc/
2. Hamilton BE, Martin JA, Ventura SJ. Births: Preliminary Data for 2007. *National Vita Statistics Reports* 57(12) Hyattsville, MD: National Center for Health Statistics, March 2009. Available at:
www.cdc.gov/nchs/data/nvsr/nvsr57/nvsr57_12.pdf
3. Levit K, Wier L, Stranges E, Ryan K, Elixhauser A. *HCUP Facts and Figures: Statistics on Hospital-based Care in the United States, 2007.* Rockville, MD: Agency for Healthcare Research and Quality, 2009. Available at: www.hcup-us.ahrq.gov/reports/factsandfigures/2007/TOC_2007.jsp
4. Russo CA, Wier L, Steiner C. Hospitalizations Related to Childbirth, 2006. Rockville, MD: Agency for Healthcare Research and Quality, 2009. (HCUP Statistical Brief, 71.) Available at:
www.hcup-us.ahrq.gov/reports/statbriefs/sb71.pdf
5. Andrews RM. The National Hospital Bill: The Most Expensive Conditions by Payer, 2006. Rockville, MD: Agency for Healthcare Research and Quality, 2008. (HCUP Statistical Brief, 59.) Available at:
www.hcup-us.ahrq.gov/reports/statbriefs/sb59.pdf

be liberated- from pain and perceived risk, to being drugged during their baby's births. The painlessness vs. the increased adverse effects to mothers and babies has been glossed over for the sake of an institutional status quo and for profit. The number of maternal deaths and infant deaths from our health care system in the US is a shocking testament to how interference with the natural order of things can take a dramatic toll on our current and future well-being.

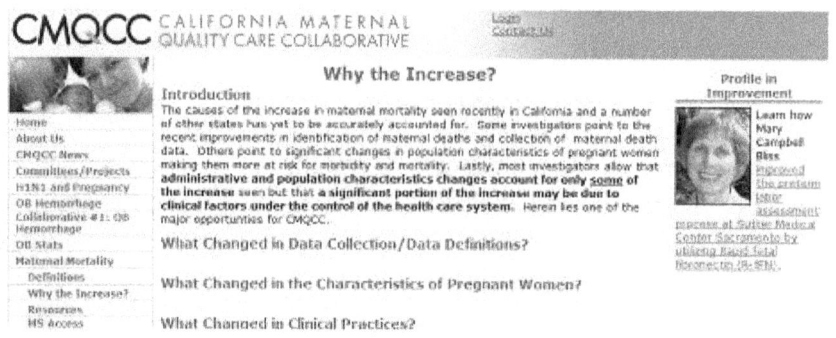

"These are rare events. They serve as a canary in the mine shaft, they tell us that we need to look more carefully at the *system of maternity care*. Overall, childbirth is very safe. This is a national disgrace and a call to action."

Dr. Elliot Main, Chairman,
Chief of Obstetrics at California Pacific Medical Center in San Francisco

In 1985 my daughter was born at a birth center with the new version of a midwife in California, Certified Nurse Midwife. We did a major remodel of our house while I was pregnant with her.

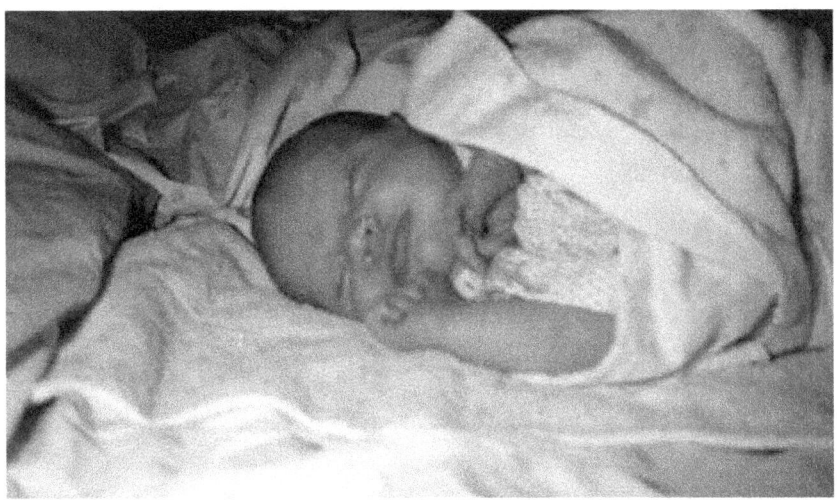

My daughter, just born, in 1985

She grew up in a house built in the 1950's, and we did another major remodeling while living in that house. She would have ingested lead dust from the paints released during the remodeling, as lead was not banned in house interior paint until 1970 in the US. Our house is very close to the main artery into our town: we breathe the fumes from the 24 hour car traffic which contains methylmercury[17]-a persistent version of mercury that gets into our air and water.

---

[17] http://www.usgs.gov/themes/factsheet/146-00/

## The Mercury Cycle

The mercury cycle

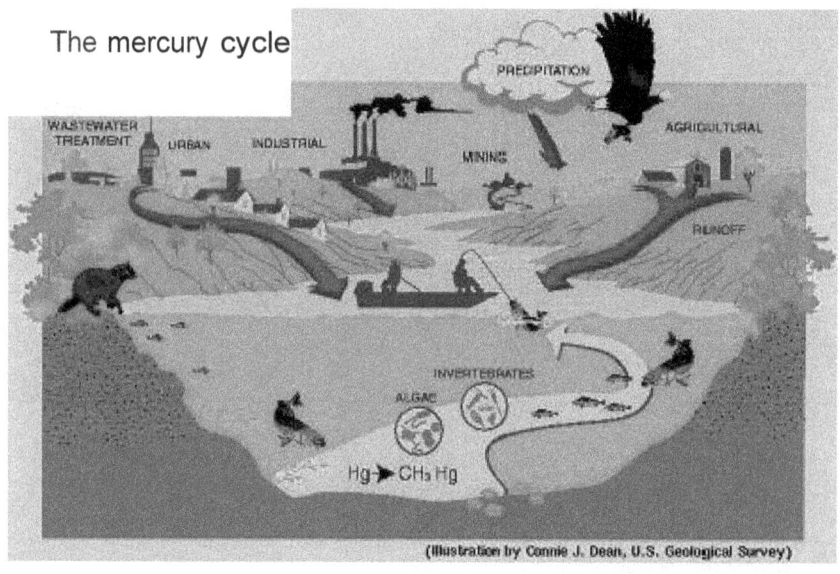

(Illustration by Connie J. Dean, U.S. Geological Survey)

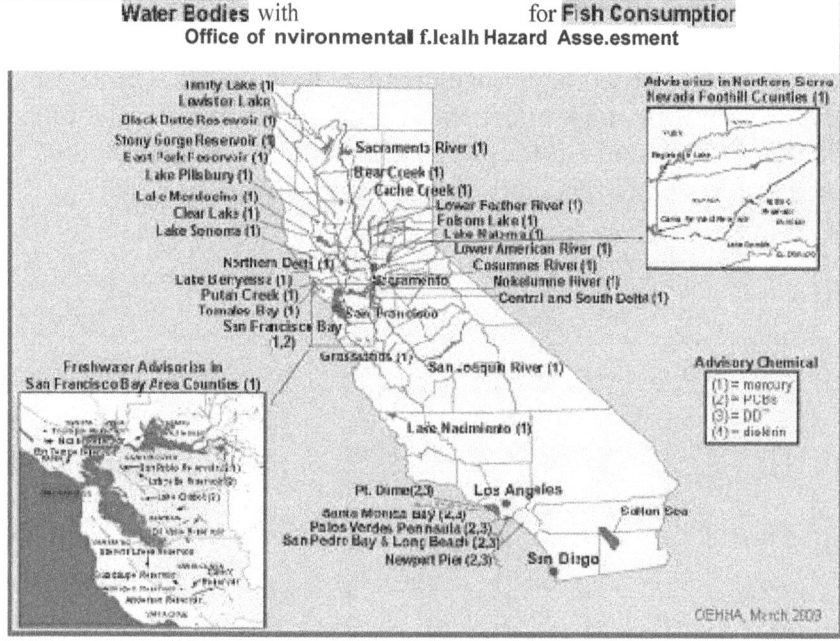

She ate the food I prepared for her, chock full of pesticides, PBDE's and PCBs. I know there were a lot of pesticides on our vegetables and fruit, I did not know that BPA, a hormone disruptor, was in the cans, in the vinyl lunch box she took to school and in the storage containers we used which have been associated with thyroid disease, obesity and diabetes, endometriosis, uterine fibroids and infertility, and immune-related disease, such as asthma or allergies. We lived on cheese and tortillas and pizza. And fish sticks- our favorite! Damn the mercury that is in the fish I fed my children for so many years.

We loved our hamburgers and spaghetti too- wow, hormone growth promoters[18] were in our beef and I did not know that early exposure for my daughter could change her gene environment which may basically re-program her body's resilience, reproduction and metabolism later in life. And she would not get nutrients from the processed foods and genetically modified fake foods that I fed her like Cheetos and Cheerios. Recently an article came out with research showing that GMO toxins are in babies in utero[19]. The altering of the very foundational components of our lives, the poisoning of our food, -our seeds and soil – the free gifts of our Mother Earth- really gave me pause, because I learned that we could be compromising the structural integrity of our bodies and bones and brains by this, and inadvertently passing it onto two generations of our beloved children and grandchildren.

And I did not know that flame retardants were in our sofas, which are called perchlorates and currently found in many commonly consumed foods and beverages, including lettuce, milk and produce, according to FDA data. This hormone disruptor can impede the iodine needed by the thyroid, which can have an effect on early brain and nervous system development in fetuses and children. Mother's breast milk can concentrate this chemical and it can be passed onto nursing infants. "Most of the toxic pentaBDE ever made is still in furniture inside our homes and schools," Penta-BDE contamination of the environment is a "chemical time bomb" on a huge scale according to

---

[18] http://www.iatp.org/documents/exposure-to-exogenous-estrogens-in-food-possible-impact-on-human-development-and-health
http://www.iatp.org/documents/smart-guide-hormones-in-the-food-system
[19] http://www.ncbi.nlm.nih.gov/pubmed/21338670

**Dr. Susan Shaw,** Director of the Marine Environmental Research Institute (MERI). "Given the demonstrated toxicity of pentaBDEs, the prospect of diminished intelligence in children and reduced fertility our population looms in our not-too distant future." [20]

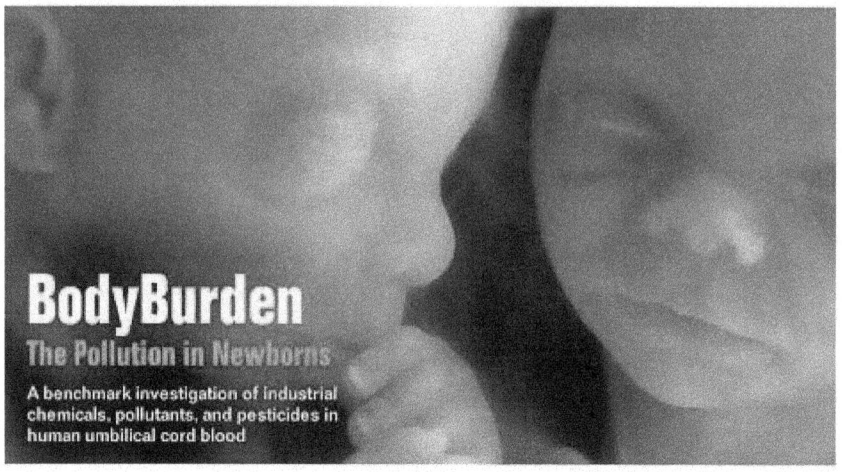

But we have been the guinea pigs.

Just an overwhelming story of increasing and ubiquitous modern hazards in our lives. I felt like I was in a Greek tragedy and wanted to poke out my eyes like Oedipus, so I would not see the horror of this situation and my role in it. I felt adulterated personally and had to know more about what I could do to lessen the hazards in my children's and grandchildren's lives now, where they are living in San Francisco's Parkside Neighborhood.

I bought some simple kits at Cole Hardware on Polk Street and tested their rental house's water and interior paint. I checked the water report, there is chloramine and fluoride added to it,(which is not a great thing for a pregnant woman to drink), but generally the San Francisco Hetch Hetchy water from the Sierra is pure enough to not warrant special reports to the EPA. [21]

---

[20] http://healthychild.org/blog/comments/toxic_flame_retardants_manufactured_by_chemtura_may_have_caused_massive_har/
[21] http://sfwater.org/modules/showdocument.aspx?documentid=1064

I found specific neighborhood info on an EPA site, that the local elementary school where my grandchildren would be attending, was found to have lead-penetrated soil from the old school's paint that was torn down and replaced. I want to test their house garden soils now too, before they start growing their own food there. [22]

I learned so much more about the history of birth in the US, and its sordid story.[23] Are we even given the freedom of choice on how we may want to birth in our technological, corporatized birthing practices today?

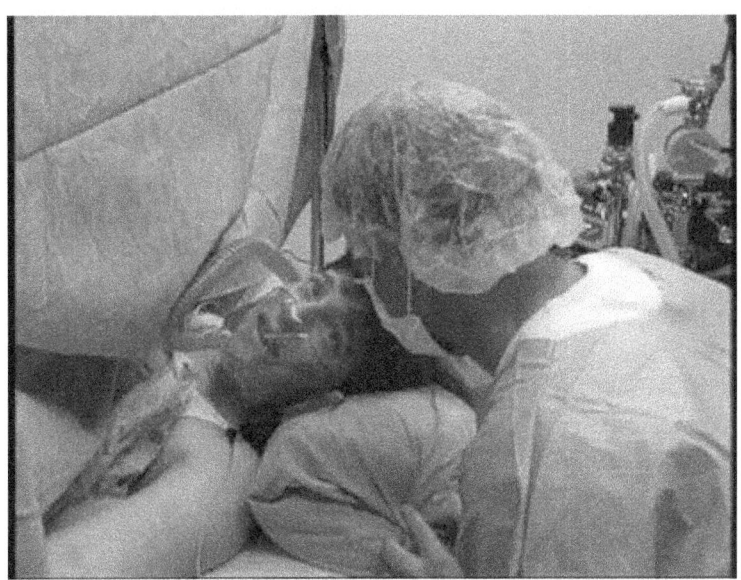

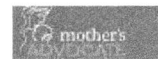

There are too many interventions to the most natural development of human evolution- bringing life into the world. Babies are subjected to increasing numbers of cesarean section deliveries(in US+30%)[24] and antibiotics, both which seriously hinder the child's

---

[22] http://www.envirostor.dtsc.ca.gov/public/map.asp?global_id=38820001
[23] http://www.ourbodiesourselves.org/book/companion.asp?id=21&compID=75
http://midwiferytoday.com/articles/timeline.asp
http://www.injoyvideos.com/mothersadvocate/videos.html
[24] http://www.oecd-ilibrary.org/social-issues-migration-health/health-at-a-glance-2011/caesarean-sections_health_glance-2011-37-en;jsessionid=2wn97opa9t8cj.delta

ability to culture the essential flora in its gut. These children are at a higher risk of developing allergies and asthma later down the road, as well as other chronic conditions, including ADHD and autism.[25] I worried that we had so altered our body's natural capabilities, that we may have even compromised our body's ability to birth. I realized very personally that we embody the ravages that we are perpetrating on the Earth, our Mother Earth, who gives us her free gifts of air and water and soil. We have corrupted these gifts and now they are us, our bodies and legacy. There is no gated neighborhood to which we can retreat for protection from modern life's polluted air, water or soil.

I am a grandmother now, of twin girls.

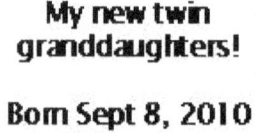

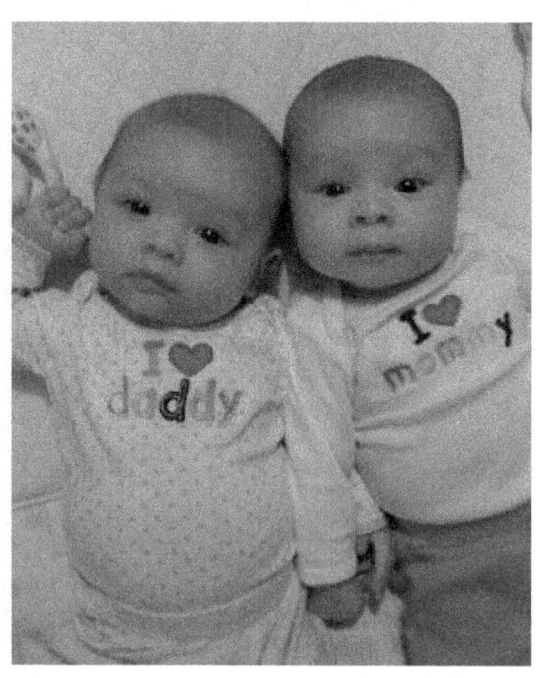

I found it hard to wait for their arrival. I did not have the same physical, embodied relationship with them that I had with my own two children, yet my feeling for them is intense and emotional. Our relationship is immutable and life-changing for me. I knew that their life force was growing in the dark, protective womb of their mother-

---

[25] http://www.environmentalhealthnews.org/ehs/newscience/2011/11/2011-1114-c-section-ups-asthma-at-three/

which contained all that they needed. But I knew from pulling together this story of my environmental lineage and legacy, that they could be influenced by outside forces, not by the conscious will of their mother, nor by any truly rational choices of our culture, but just as immutably, by me and my ancestor's personal actions, choices and ignorance. I realize that how I live on this earth is what my granddaughters will inherit. Their changeable physiology creates a responsibility on me, because I would never want an action that I do to harm my grandchildren. I understand that my relationship with my all-encompassing Mother Earth somehow is immutable too, just like my relationship with my granddaughters. And I feel that my Mother Earth who holds and nurtures me and feeds me is beneficent. She would not want to harm either, yet she accepts what is happening to her, with involuntary surrender. I live within and enable the perpetuation of a system that harms our world and our babies.

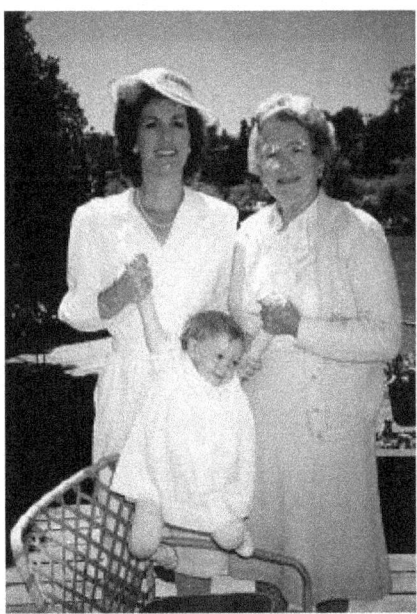

This became an existential dilemma for me. How do I live in the real world, hold to the faith and conviction I have in the beneficence of our existence and not drop into despair and hopelessness?

The word EcoBirth came to me in the midst of this search, it has come to integrate many strands in my life- my feminine qualities, living a faith-based life, connecting to my lineage, unique to place and time in San Francisco, and my primary, immutable, relationship with Mother Earth. I want to take responsibility for the shape that our world is in now, by seeing the hope and love that is needed to enable the next generations to heal it. I do not have the answers for them, but I can try to hold the space to allow them to find those answers, by seeing the truth of what is happening now, processing it in my heart and naming it in public. I see birth as the metaphor for transformation and creation that if honored, will create a paradigm shift in our culture's consciousness.

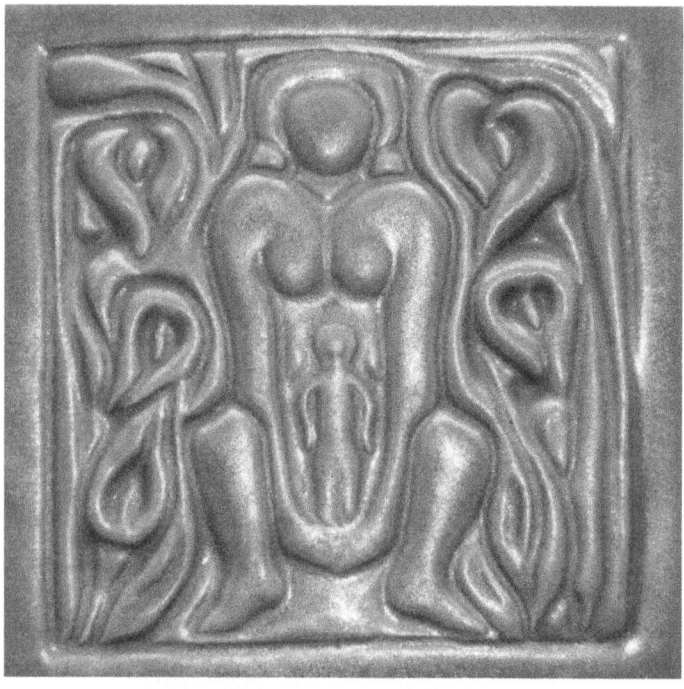

And that consciousness would realize that we are all related, that our planet home is an extraordinarily perfect balance of natural cycles and that caring for our one natural life will enable us all to be well. That we are caught in a web of a story that separates us, gives us a false sense that we are independent, alone and in charge of our own destiny, with no need for anyone else. Disconnected, unrelated, isolated. Not true.

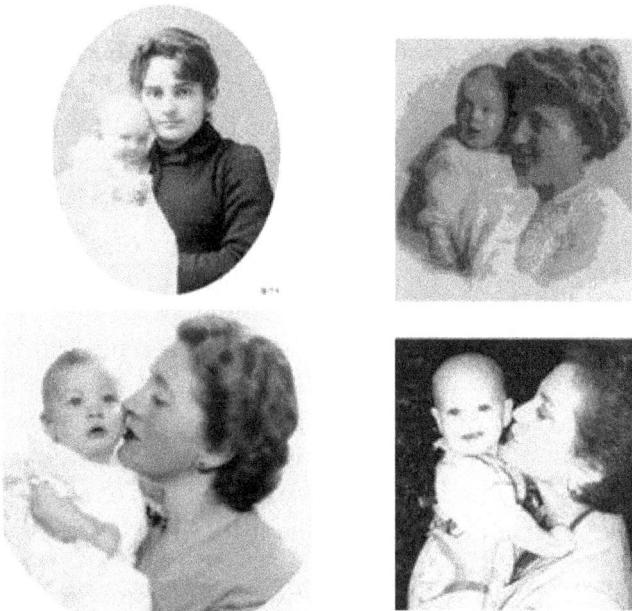

Our true story is about the extraordinary connection in ourselves that goes all the way back to the first stirring of life gathered on this earth.

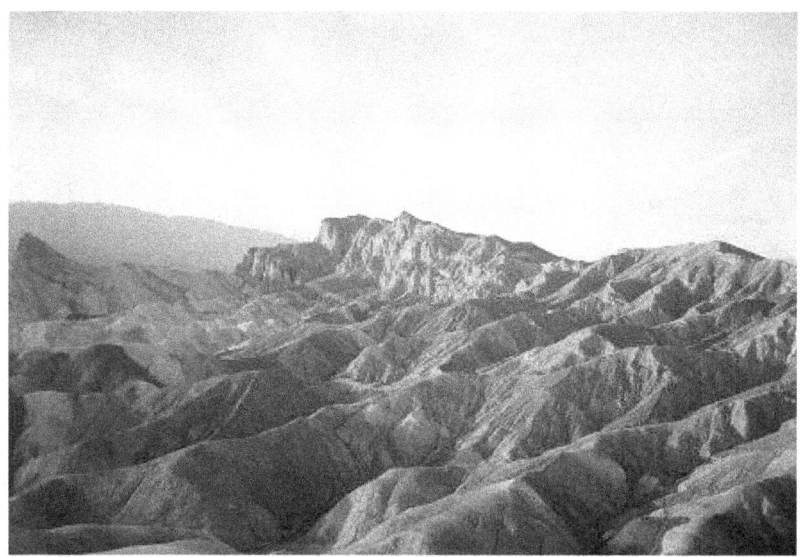

The first law of ecology is that everything is related to everything else.
-Barry Commoner

We were born from our mothers, they were born from their mothers, and we were formed from bits of their bodies all the way back to the first amoeba- there is still a small bit of that life spark in us. We could not be here without all this lineage and heritage; we are dependent on their living and giving. It is a wonderful story of relationship based on love and compassion, unbreakable, freely given.

We have just lost our connection to our Mother Earth and to ourselves and our fellow kin, but becoming aware that we are all in the same interdependent living system is hopeful, faithful and so biologically real. We have since the beginning of time, given our feminine, maternal gifts to our children, with no thought for payment. That instinct for offering ourselves will be found again-to reclaim our rightful place in the order of life. We are not lost or truly harmful to our following generations, we are their life-givers.

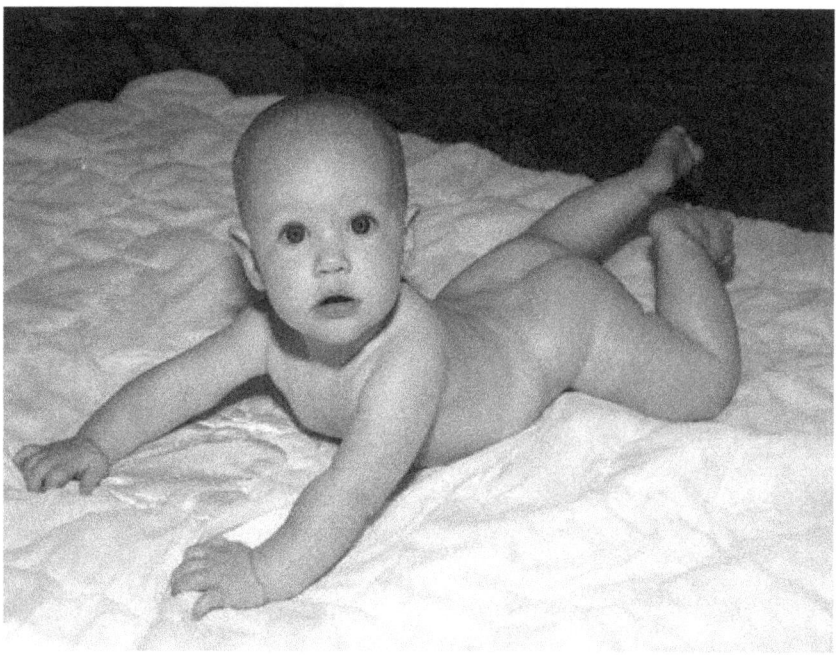

I know that that wicker crib was a hard and tangible part of my inheritance and my legacy to my children; I know that that Chanel #5 is still on my bureau, symbolizing all the love given and harm perpetrated; I sleep next to it every night. But I chose to see the respect and acknowledgment that my mother was giving me when she gave me that meaningful gift. And I chose to work with a fierce passion to make right this world for my grandchildren, and your grandchildren. I trust in my connection to my mother and grandmother, and I see my relationship to all kin in our world, on our earth, in our cosmos, with a gaze of love and compassion. I look to receive that gaze in return, with an open, wounded heart, vulnerable and strong.

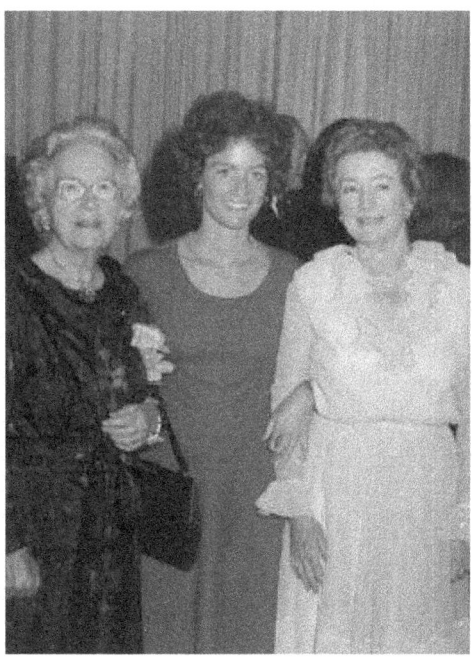

I just heard of research that said that a mother's laughter makes her breast milk healthier for her child- - there is really nothing more miraculous than that! We can change the world with love and laughter and it will respond with health, happiness and true acceptance of our rightful place in it.[26]

---

[26] http://holistic-healing4all.blogspot.com/2008/06/mothers-laughter-makes-breast-milk.html

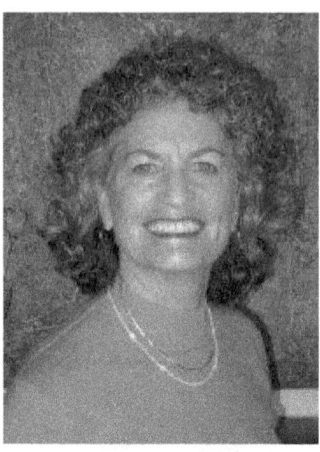

## About Molly

Molly McGettigan Arthur is a native San Franciscan; she graduated from UC Berkeley and has had extensive experience working with startups and growing networks in her professional sales career. She has sold media, software and sponsorships for the premier internet trade show and is currently selling software products to election bureaus in the western states. She and her husband of 38 years have raised two children in Marin County and happily her new twin granddaughters live close by in San Francisco! She is the inspiration behind EcoBirth whose vision is -*Relating earth and birth- caring for one natural life so we will all be well*. She has a fierce desire to protect all our children and grandchildren and fully appreciate the freely given gifts of our Mother Earth. She sees birth as the metaphor for transformation and creation that if honored, will create a paradigm shift in our culture's consciousness. Her focus is on inspiring women to change our culture's story to compassion for the environments of Earth and Birth and to impel social change to sustain healthy, caring humans and a healed earth home.
http://www.ecobirthgreenwomb.org

# About The Author

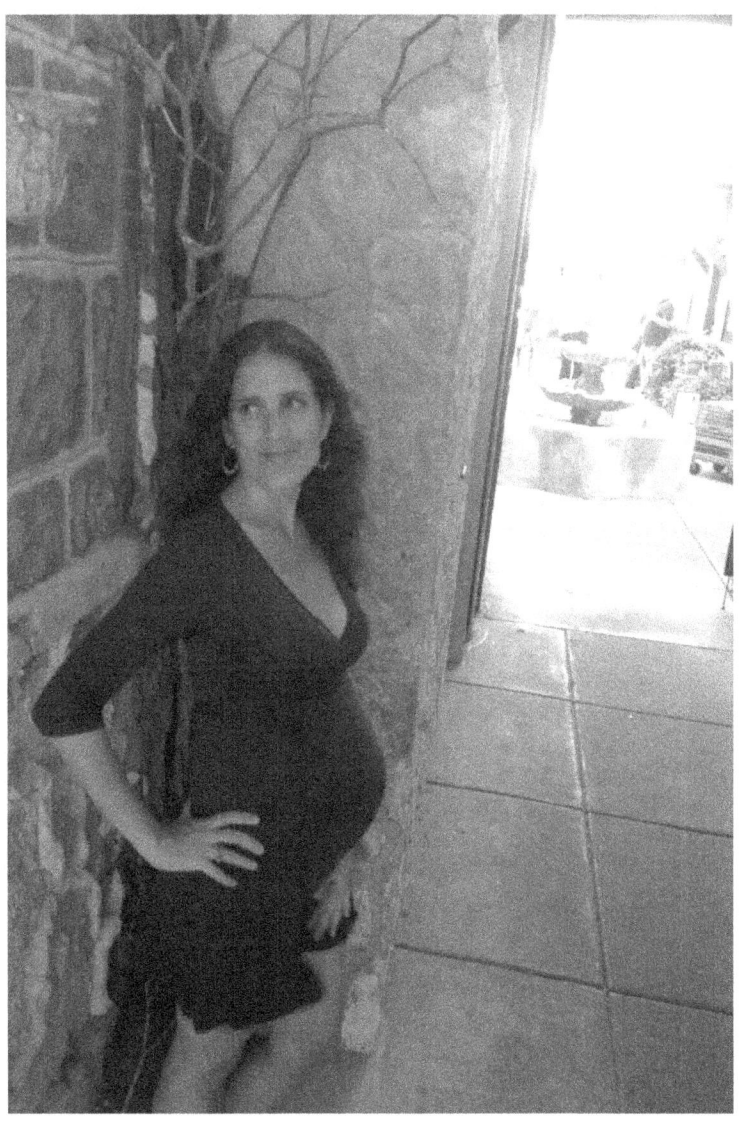

**Mary Oscategui** is an international business consultant and holistic educator who specializes in maternal health, fitness, nutrition, sleep and green living. Mary is a leader in educational development and has been consulting and guiding hundreds of clients for the last 17 years.

She is the *Founder, CEO,* and *President* of the International Maternity Institute (IMI), International Academy of Baby Planner Professionals (IABPP), TheBabyPlanner.Com, and Co-Founder and Executive Director of the Association of Professional Sleep Consultants (APSC). Additionally Mary also offers health and fitness services through Physical Awakening.com, a holistic integrative approach offering the services of yoga, meditation, pilates, fitness, and nutrition. She is the author of *The Baby Planner Profession: What You Need to Know!* and her latest book, *Green Body Green Birth*.

Mary's work in the health, fitness, and maternity industry is backed up by a multitude of prestigious certifications. She is a writer, speaker, educator, coach, baby planner, stress management coach, wellness coach, sleep consultant, certified yoga and pilates instructor, certified personal trainer, holistic nutrition consultant, going green consultant, greenproofer, and birthing options advocate.

Mary enjoys empowering, educating, and supporting expectant and new parents to know all their options so that they may confidently make informed decisions for themselves and their family in the healthiest and safest way. Mary also advises and coaches maternity professionals offering a wealth of knowledge and support. Her enthusiasm, inspiration, creativity, and knowledge has helped launch many maternity start-up businesses in 22 countries around the world.

Mary introduced a new approach to the baby planning industry by focusing on the needs of her clients through parental education and emotional support and established the first and only certification program currently in the baby planning industry.

Most recently Mary has been working to raise the bar for the child sleep consulting industry by expanding a sleep consultant's role to include working with expecting families, setting forth a formal definition, standards of practice and boundaries to practice for the sleep consulting profession via the IMI Maternity & Child Sleep Consultant Certification.

Mary is mother to four year old, "Bella Luna" and is currently expecting her second child, "Taj Orion Sky", in August 2012. She is fluent in Spanish and resides in Marin, California with her family.

*Resources*

**GREEN ORGANIZATIONS:**

Environmental Working Group (EWG)

Healthy Child/Healthy World

Making Our Milk Safe (MOMS)

Children's Environmental Health Network (CEHN)

Center for Children's Health & the Environment (CCHE)

Council on Environmental Health

Institute for Children's Environmental Health (ICEH)

ECOBIRTH-Women for Earth and Birth

WHO Children's Environmental Health

Agency for Toxic Substances & Disease Registry

The Natural Child Project

Every Mother Counts

Ava Anderson Non-Toxic

Coalition for Improving Maternity Services

Children's Health Environmental Coalition

Campaign For Safe Cosmetics

Good Guide

Earth911

Global Footprint Network (Ecofoot)

Friends of the Earth International

Earth Island Institute

The Safe Playgrounds Project

EPA Office of Children's Health Protection

World Wildlife Fund: Global Toxic Initiative

Alvepalmas.org

Bioneers

Cali Bamboo

Care2

Coop America

Green Business Bureau

Green America

Greenguard

Rainforest Alliance

Biodegradable Products Institute (BPI)

CampaignEarth

Earth Screen

EarthShare.org

GoGreenNow.net

Root Systems Institute

TreeHugger.com

World Watch Institute

World Wildlife Fund

GreenPeace

EarthJustice

GreenCorps

AddedValue

Green Plus: Institute for Sustainable Development

The Conservation Fund

EcoTrust

Natural Resource Defense Council

National Geographic Society

**GREEN PREGNANCY BOOKS**

The Complete Organic Pregnancy by Deirdre Dolan and Alexandra Zissu

Raising Baby Green: The Earth-Friendly Guide to Pregnancy, Childbirth, and Baby Care by Alan Greene, Jeanette Pavini and Theresa Foy DiGeronimo

The Green Pregnancy Diet: Healthy eating habits for mommy, baby and the planet by Radha McLean

A Green Guide to Your Natural Pregnancy and Birth: The Kind Way for You, Your Baby, and the Environment by Claire Gill

Green Guide Families: The Complete Reference for Eco-Friendly Parents The Everything Green Baby Book: From pregnancy to baby's first year - an easy and affordable guide to help you care for your baby - and for the earth! by Jenn Savedge

Green Baby by Susannah Marriott

Green Fertility: Nature's Secrets For Making Babies: A Powerful Proven Plan To Help You Get Pregnant Fast & Have a Healthy Baby by Niels H Lauersen and Colette Bouchez

Growing Up Green: Baby and Child Care: Volume 2 in the Bestselling Green This! Series by Deirdre Imus

The Eco-nomical Baby Guide: Down-to-Earth Ways for Parents to Save Money and the Planet by Joy Hatch and Rebecca Kelley

Baby Greens: A Live-Food Approach for Children of All Ages by Michaela Lynn

Smart Mama's Green Guide: Simple Steps to Reduce Your Child's Toxic Chemical Exposure by Jennifer Taggart

Green Fertility: Nature's Secrets For Making Babies: A Powerful Proven Plan To Help You Get Pregnant Fast & Have a Healthy Baby by Niels H. Lauersen and Colette Bouchez

Heart and Hands: A Midwife's Guide to Pregnancy and Birth by Elizabeth Davis, Linda Harrison and Suzanne Arms

Imperfectly Natural Baby and Toddler: How to Be a Green Parent in Today's Busy World by Janey Lee Grace

Green Kids, Sage Families: The Ultimate Guide to Raising Your Organic Kids by Lynda Fassa and Vanessa Williams

Mother's Little Helper - an old fashioned guide to raising your baby chemical-free by Wendyl Nissen

Healthy From Day 1 Create Your Baby's Healthiest Nursery by Justin Valley

Child Health Guide: Holistic Pediatrics for Parents by Randall Neustaedter

Teach Yourself Green Parenting (Teach Yourself - General) by Lynoa Cattanach

Baby Green by Jill Barker

Natural Hospital Birth: The Best of Both Worlds (Non) by Cynthia Gabriel

Natural Childbirth the Bradley Way: Revised Edition by Susan McCutcheon-Rosegg, Erick Ingraham, Robin Yoko Burningham and Robert A. Bradley

Natural Birth: A Holistic Guide to Pregnancy, Childbirth, and Breastfeeding by Kristina Turner

Active Birth : The New Approach to Giving Birth Naturally, Revised Edition (Non) by Janet Balaskas

Your Best Birth: Know All Your Options, Discover the Natural Choices, and Take Back the Birth Experience by Ricki Lake, Abby Epstein and Jacques Moritz

Adventures in Natural Childbirth: Tales from Women on the Joys, Fears, Pleasures, and Pains of Giving Birth Naturally by Janet Schwegel and Pam England

A Wise Birth: Bringing Together the Best of Natural Childbirth and Modern Medicine by Penny Armstrong, Sheryl Feldman and Sheila Kitzinger

Husband-Coached Childbirth (Fifth Edition): The Bradley Method of Natural Childbirth by Robert A. Bradley, Marjie Hathaway, Jay Hathaway and James Hathaway

HypnoBirthing: The Mongan Method: A natural approach to a safe, easier, more comfortable birthing (3rd Edition) by Marie F. Mongan and Lorne R. Campbell

The Natural Pregnancy Book: Herbs, Nutrition, and Other Holistic Choices by Aviva Jill Romm M.D. and Ina May Gaskin

Painless Childbirth: An Empowering Journey Through Pregnancy and Childbirth by Giuditta Tornetta

Calm Birth: New Method for Conscious Childbirth by Robert Newman and David Chamberlain

A Labour Of Love: A Guide To Natural Childbirth Without Fear by Gabrielle Targett

Natural Health after Birth: The Complete Guide to Postpartum Wellness by Aviva Jill Romm

Your Non-Toxic Pregnancy by Susannah Marriott

Easy Green Living: The Ultimate Guide to Simple, Eco-Friendly Choices for You and Your Home by Renée Loux

Living Organic: Easy Steps to an Organic Lifestyle by Helen Porter; Helen Quested; Patricia Thomas; Editor-Adrienne Clarke

The Yoga of Birth By Katie Manitsas

The Sacred Nature of Birth By KaRa Maria Ananda

Green Guide Families: The Complete Reference for Eco-Friendly Parents by Catherine Zandonella

**GREEN PREGNANCY WEBSITES**

Safecosmetics.org

Ewg.org

Goodguide.com

Safemilk.org

Natural Parenting

GreenWaLa.com

NaturalNews.com

Natural Baby Pros

The Unneceserean.com

GreenFertility.com

Midwifery Today

Greenmommy.ca

EcoMom.com

FoodHasPower.com

CompletelyNourished.org

DrMomma.org

BirthYourWay.org

PracticeGreenHealth.org

GrowingGreenBaby.com

PracticallyGreen.com

TheDailyGreen.com

MindBodyGreen.com

Rodale.com

SinsofGreenwashing.com

GreenOptions.com

TheGreenMama.com

TheGreenGirls.com

TheGreenMomReview.com

GreenandCleanmom.org

OrganicMania.com

Greenmomsmeet.com

moregreenmoms.com

naturemoms.com

happygreenbabies.com

greenmomspreventdisease.com

greenmomstoday.com

mindfulmomma.com

livegreenmom.com

**GREEN NUTRITION BOOKS**

Feeding Baby Green: The Earth Friendly Program for Healthy, Safe Nutrition During Pregnancy, Childhood, and Beyond by Alan R. Greene

Toxic Free by Debra Lynn Dadd

Eating for Pregnancy: The Essential Nutrition Guide and Cookbook for Today's Mothers-to-Be by Catherine Jones and Rose Ann Hudson

The 100 Healthiest Foods to Eat During Pregnancy: The Surprising Unbiased Truth about Foods You Should be Eating During Pregnancy but Probably Aren't by Jonny Bowden Ph.D. C.N.S. and Allison Tannis MS

The Green Pregnancy Diet: Healthy eating habits for mommy, baby and the planet by Radha McLean

The Well-Rounded Pregnancy Cookbook: Give Your Baby a Healthy Start with 100 Recipes That Adapt to Fit How You Feel byKaren Gurwitz and Jen Hoy

Green for Life by Victoria Boutenko and A. William Menzin M.D

The Healthy Green Drink Diet: Advice and Recipes to Energize, Alkalize, Lose Weight, and Feel Great by Jason Manheim

The Complete Idiot's Guide to Plant-Based Nutrition by Julieanna Hever M.S., R.D., C.P.T.

Green Smoothie Revolution: The Radical Leap Towards Natural Health by Victoria Boutenko

The Little Green Book of Nutrition: 250 Tips for an Eco Lifestyle (Little Green Books) by Diane Millis

The Green Foods Bible: Everything You Need to Know about Barley Grass, Wheatgrass, Kamut, Chlorella, Spirulina and More by David Sandova

The Complete Idiot's Guide to Organic Living by Eliza Sarasohn and Sonia Weiss

Nutrition for Healthy Living by Wendy Schiff

Clean, Green, and Lean: Get Rid of the Toxins That Make You Fat by Walter Crinnion

Rainbow Green Live-Food Cuisine by Gabriel Cousens

Organic Living by Michael Van Straten

Going Green 101: A Guide To Organic Living by Gregory Branson-Trent

It's Easy Being Green: A Handbook for Earth-Friendly Living by Crissy Trask

Living Green for Health by Jr. Paul Yanick

Everything You Need to Know About Green Living by Diane Gow McDilda

The Yoga of Eating: Transcending Diets and Dogma to Nourish the Natural Self by Charles Eisenstein

The Yoga of Nutrition by Omraam Mikhael Aivanhov

**GREEN MAGAZINES**

Kiwi

Green Child

Green Parent

Green Lifestyle

Organic Lifestyle

Living Green

Mothering

Mother Earth News

Boho

Organic Spa Magazine

Natural Living

Natural Health

Natural Home and Garden

## GREENPROOFERS & GREENBIRTH EDUCATORS
Links to Businesses can be found by visiting the International Maternity Institute at MaternityInstitute.com

**US Greenproofer & Greenbirth Educators**
**Mill Valley, CA**
Mary Oscategui
Emily Schaffer

**Pasadena, California**
Heather Crummer Engemann

**Phoenix, AZ**
Tonya Sackowicz
Heather Newton

**Beverly Hills, CA**
Jennifer Yozamp

**Los Angeles, CA**
Saray Hill

**Orange County, CA**
Heather Newton
Denise Xagorarakis

**Denver, Colorado**
Annie Mullens

**Fort Collins, Colorado**
Sarah Cody

**Coral Springs, FL**
Danielle Corradino

**Longwood, FL**
Jennifer Rumsey

**Orlando, FL**
Adriana Babler
Jessica Wilson

**Franklin, IN**
Cortney Gibson

**Richmond, Maine**
Tiffany Carter

**St Louis, MO**
Nicole Hatchet
Deborah Zorensky
Anya Kaufman

**Rochester, NY**
Adriana Lozada

**New York, NY**
Yolanda Allen

**Cleveland, Ohio**
Tiffany Sumner

**Parma, Ohio**
Sara Szelagowski

**Providence, RI**
Alicia Kamm

**Katy, TX**
Sherri Levinton

**Houston, TX**
Nina Bassett

**Pharr, TX**
Nancy Cavazos

**Manassas, VA**
Michelle Winters

**Wisconsin**
Amanda Hammond

**International Greenproofer & GreenBirth Educators**

**Argentina**
Mariela Seijo
Claudia Cubilla Rocha

**Australia**
Sally de Hennin

**Canada**
Marie-Pier Villeneuve
Karlee Lisafeld

**Hong Kong**
Sarah Sanesi
Coco Wong

**Italy**
Michela Fratus

**Germany**
Veronique Goldbrunner

**Singapore**
Constance Chiang
Coco Wong

www.ingramcontent.com/pod-product-compliance
Lightning Source LLC
Chambersburg PA
CBHW051756040426
42446CB00007B/401